The Healing Power of Jerusalem Artichoke Fiber

 Enhance the Healing Response of Antibiotics...

 Improve Your Gastrointestinal & Immune Health...

 Normalize Blood Sugar Levels...

 Maximize Your Energy Levels & Vitality...

 ...WITH THE MIRACLE OF PLANT PREBIOTICS

by Michael Loes, M.D., M.D.(H.)

The Healing Power of Jerusalem Artichoke Fiber

Disclaimer: The material in this presentation is for informational purposes only and not intended for the treatment or diagnosis of individual disease. Please, visit a qualified medical or other health professional for specifically diagnosing any ailments mentioned or discussed in detail in this material.

This information is presented by independent scientific and medical experts whose sources of information include studies from the world's medical and scientific literature, clinical and anecdotal reports, and the doctors' personal experiences with family, friends, and patients.

ISBN 1-893910-09-1

First Printing, December 2000
Published by Freedom Press
1801 Chart Trail
Topanga, CA 90290

Bulk Orders Available: (310) 455-2995
E-mail: info@freedompressonline.com
or sales@freedompressonline.com

Acknowledgements

I WISH TO ACKNOWLEDGE the important contributions of the following persons for their insights in the writing of this book: Rudolf Kunze, Ph.D., for his expertise on the benefits of inulin; Dr. Monike Krüger for her insights into the beneficial effects of inulin; Joachim Solfronk of Symbio Pharm GmbH for his tremendous insights on the importance of healthy bacterial populations and for insight on the quality of commercial probiotic products; Adel Joanne Spangler for secretarial assistance; Neil Cohen for his research prowess; Joachim Lehmann for his insight in the structuring and simplifying of this book; and, of course, my patients for seeking natural healing pathways. I also offer my heartfelt gratitude to David William Steinman, M.A., for his unparalleled editorial and publishing skills and much-appreciated assistance in getting my work out to the public.

Table of Contents

Foreword

AS A HEALTH JOURNALIST with a young child, I am always on the look-out for ways to improve my family's resistance to illness and minimize our need for doctor visits. That's why I became so excited when I learned about the many uses of a non-digestible sugar with a sweet pleasant taste that is extracted from the root of the Jerusalem artichoke.

As someone with years of experience in reporting on health issues, I count inulin as one of the major breakthroughs in dietary supplements in recent years. Inulin addresses many important health issues that can help to make both adults and children healthier and more resistant to both acute infectious illness as well as long-term health problems including cancer and diabetes, both increasing at alarming rates among members of our generation and that of our children's generation.

When adults and children are prone to chronic infectious illnesses, it is likely they are frequently being prescribed antibiotics. Make no mistake. The use of antibiotics is necessary and good. However, we also know that high dosages of antibiotics and especially those with a broad spectrum of action, including the tetracyclines, destroy both harmful and beneficial bacteria that reside in the gastrointestinal tract.

As we are beginning to recognize only belatedly, beneficial bacteria are critical to both adult and children's health. Beneficial bacteria help to assimilate nutrients and produce key vitamins as well as stimulate various immune functions that enable our bodies to resist both acute and chronic diseases. There is no question that healthy populations of beneficial bacteria in our gastrointestinal system play a crucial role in maintaining over-all health. What I find so pleasing and important about *Inulin: The Antibiotic Companion* is that author Michael Loes, M.D., M.D.(H.) does such an excellent job of detailing the multi-faceted beneficial impact of beneficial bacteria on overall human health—for both children and adults. He also does a great job of sharing with the health-conscious public his knowledge of *prebiotics*: that is, feeding or fertilizing the ben-eficial bacteria in the gastrointestinal tract to insure their healthy population.

Inulin, which is completely safe and without any drug interactions whatsoever, offers both adults and children an important method of cultivating healthy intestinal flora. Inulin is a premiere prebiotic, which means that these non-digestible complex sugars are taken up intact in the gut where they serve as food for our most valuable, friendly strains of bacterial microorganisms, helping to establish the proper balance of beneficial intestinal flora. As such, a *prebiotic* serves as "food" for beneficial bacteria in the colon.

A healthy intestine in both children and adults contains bil-lions of friendly bacteria—including up to 400 different

 ## Prebiotic

**CYBER
INSIGHT**

Definition:

... a non digestible food ingredient that beneficially affects the host by selectively stimulating the growth and/or activity of one of more of the beneficial flora on the colon.

species. Incredibly, the body's beneficial bacteria outnumber the cells of the body by one-hundred fold!

These friendly bacteria are our first line of immune defense. They displace and fight off unfriendly bacteria and internal fungi that can set the stage for both adult and childhood illness. They even increase the body's levels of interferon, a mighty immune-boosting hormone.

This is all very critical to our health. If harmful bacteria propagate and gain the upper hand, we will not only be prone to infectious disease but our bodies will produce toxic, carcinogenic substances. We will also suffer constipation and diarrhea.

But here's the problem that adults—and children especially—face as they grow up in a toxic world. Stress, medications and poor diet reduce friendly bacteria even further, leaving them even more vulnerable to disease. Antibiotics can be the biggest culprits in destroying our friendly bacteria. At high dosages, they wipe out *all* bacteria inside the child's body, the good along with the bad.

Once that happens, the race is on as to which microorganisms, the good guys or the bad guys, set up shop in that empty real estate inside yours or your child's gut.

Even if we don't take antibiotics, we almost certainly consume them in animal products. Over 35 million pounds of antibiotics are produced in the U.S. each year, and animals are given the vast bulk of them. Cattle, pigs and poultry are routinely given big helpings of antibiotics to prevent infections from spreading in their stressful, crowded quarters. In Western Europe, giving antibiotics to cattle is outlawed, as is the importation of American beef; this is, in part, due to all the antibiotics fed to U.S. cattle.

This is why we must be extra careful to replenish and stabilize friendly bacteria in the gastrointestinal tract. Inulin is the main food that makes friendly intestinal bacteria thrive. Now, when adults or children take inulin together with their antibiotics and following antibiotic therapy, they are providing their gut with the necessary help to enable their friendly bacteria to multiply by the millions and thrive. In essence, when we help ourselves in this way, we have positioned on our side a massive army of health defenders in our intestines that is ever on guard to protect our health.

Now readers can see why I am so excited about inulin. When consumers are prescribed antibiotics either for short or longer periods, I truly believe that they should also consider the use of inulin concurrently to maintain and replenish their population of beneficial bacteria. By doing so, they will have gone a long way towards having all of the friendly bacteria they need to keep their intestines clean, healthy and populated with a strong front line of defense to support immune function and overall health.

Be well!

David Steinman, M.A.
September 29, 2000

INTRODUCTION:

Inulin—An Exciting Health Breakthrough

AS A STUDENT OF TRADITIONAL MEDICAL education at the University of Minnesota, the gastrointestinal tract was discussed as one of the many "systems" that make-up the human body. Surely, it was stressed, that it is an important part, but under-stressed was the role it plays in balancing the body's immune defense system. The gut, for all intents and purposes, was a digestive organ.

Even through my residency in Internal Medicine at the University of Arizona in Tucson, nothing of substance was presented to reshape that view.

Now, we know considerably more. My interest has become solidly entrenched in what is now known as "integrative" or "complementary" medicine. This means that we must know and use what is useful and healthful from nutritional medicine and other holistic disciplines to help us enhance the healing response of our patients.

For years, I have prescribed healthy supplies of yogurt, acidophilus, and lactobacilli supplements for my patients requiring antibiotics. Through these, we have usually considerably shortened the term of therapy. After all, what we want is to "get the upper hand on the illness" and let the body initiate its own healing response.

Although this strategy has worked, patients' bouts with irritable bowl syndrome following their use of antibiotics persisted for days and even weeks.

My presumably non-infected patients would come in complaining of weakness, gas, bloating, belching, diarrhea. They were now "out of balance." Their gastrointestinal tracts wanted to be feeling "in tune" again.

The problem was that the viable cultures of friendly bacteria were not taking hold but rather offering only temporary help. What we needed was a pathway to "feed" and rejuvenate the remaining colonies of native friendly bacteria already residing within their gastrointestinal tracts. These particular bacteria were well-adapted to the individual biochemical variability of their host—the individual patient—and could once again thrive. They simply required a "salt lick" or stimulus to growth.

With the renewed recognition of the beneficial effects of inulin therapy, we now have a simple safe and effective answer to these worries and problems. Inulin is another one of Europe's natural medicine secrets. The data is there that it works to quickly boost back the bacteria in our gastrointestinal tract to healthy levels.

The information in this book is presented to restore vitality and health to your gastrointestinal system and, in so doing, to your overall health.

What we want is to enhance the healing response. I want to help boost your health back to salubrity—a state of beautifully enviable health.

Michael W. Loes, M.D. M.D.(H.)
Board Certified in Internal Medicine

ONE

So, the Doctor Prescribed Antibiotics... Now What Do You Do?

MARA

I WANT TO TELL YOU A STORY about one of my patients, Mara.

Mara began having problems with abnormal uterine bleeding after giving birth to her third child. She also developed several medium-sized fibroids and a prolapsed uterus. She became increasingly uncomfortable with abdominal pain and constipation and was scheduled for an elective hysterectomy.

To complicate matters, Mara also had mitral valve prolapse. Thus, she received presurgical antibiotics such as Garamycin to prevent heart valve infection. During the surgery, she was given more broad-spectrum antibiotics, this time Rocephin, and, within forty-eight hours following surgery, another round of antibiotics.

Upon seeing Mara, she was nauseated and lived on intravenous sugar for the first few days following her surgery. In addition, she had been discharged with a fever and was given another round of antibiotics, this time Keflex. Her bowels were not acting normally. She was experiencing cramping, gas, and irregular stools.

When I saw Mara, I put her on an inulin-based formula and told her to take two grams three times a day. The first thing that Mara noticed was the cramping and gas went away with-

in forty-eight hours. Her strength and energy returned quickly. Her bowel function gradually returned to normal.

Without the help of inulin, it is likely that it would have taken weeks for Mara's bowels to normalize. In fact, it is quite likely that she may have ended up with repeated courses of anti-fungal therapy because of vaginal and anal itching that was just beginning to occur from yeast overgrowth.

Fortunately, we had inulin. Mara recovered uneventfully and was thankful that her physician recognized and effectively treated the imbalance problem that had occurred within her gastrointestinal flora. The solution was natural and, by enhancing the body's healing response, insured a rapid return to health.

CYBER INSIGHT

So, your doctor has prescribed a regimen of antibiotics for you or your child. You're a fan of natural medicine. You know nature's powerful pharmacy works and, for the lengthening marathon of life, is extremely important.

Do you say no to your doctor? *No! Absolutely not!*

Antibiotics are one of the most important miracle medicines of the Twentieth Century. They are absolutely necessary to vanquishing illness and restoring the healing process. When antibiotics are a medical necessity, take them. Follow your doctor's daily dosing instructions and don't stop until you've taken them for as long as he or she has instructed. But when you do need antibiotics, your best course of action may be adding a newly recognized substance, inulin, that is becoming an integral part of complementary medicine—which is the practice of health and healing that combines the best of what your doctor has to offer from mainstream medicine with the best of natural and alternative medicine.

But let's start from the beginning.

What is an antibiotic, anyway?

ANTIBIOTICS 101

Antibiotics are chemical compounds used to kill or inhibit the growth of infectious organisms. All antibiotics possess selective toxicity, meaning that they are more toxic to an invading organism than they are to the host organism (e.g., the person taking them).

Organic compounds such as crude plant extracts have been used to fight infection since ancient times. Indeed, for many years before specific antibiotic therapy became available, a combination of bed rest, healing herbs and wholesome foods was commonly used with varying effectiveness to treat infections, even tuberculosis.

So, the Doctor Prescribed Antibiotics... Now What Do You Do?

In the 19th century French chemist Louis Pasteur discovered that certain bacteria can kill anthrax bacilli. In the early 20th century, German chemist Paul Ehrlich discovered and synthesized compounds that would selectively attack an infecting organism without harming the host. In 1928, British bacteriologist Sir Alexander Fleming discovered penicillin, a derivative of the mold *Penicillium notatum*, and showed its effectiveness against many disease-producing bacteria in laboratory cultures. Penicillin, however, was not available for use until the outbreak of World War II (1939-1945) stimulated renewed research.

Since antibiotics came into general use in the 1950s, they have transformed the patterns of disease and death. As they are effective against once highly fatal diseases such as tuberculosis, pneumonia, and septicemia, it is now less likely that people will die of infectious disease such as pneumonia or influenza. Antibiotics have also been used in the treatment or prevention of fungus infection and protozoal diseases, especially malaria. We are also less likely to die from surgery since such procedures have been made more safe for us and improved because operations can be carried out without a high risk of infection.

It is important to remember that we have not conquered infectious disease. We have simply overcome some pathogens and as well created ever more terrifying, evolved forms. Unfortunately, our misuse of antibiotics, including taking them for less than the prescribed period of time, is blamed for creating such drug-resistant strains. These can then be spread to "innocent bystanders" who never took the antibiotics at all. So it is essential that we follow our doctor's recommendations and not squander these miracles of modern medicine.

Indeed, cases of new strains of age-old pathogens have emerged with fearsome consequences. For some time during the heyday of the sixties and seventies we might have thought that we had somehow gained the upper hand against the scourge of age-old infectious diseases. We haven't. Ancient diseases caused by bacterial and viral toxins as well as parasites continue to account for half of all deaths worldwide. So, really, antibiotics are more essential to our health than ever before. The ultimate conquest of infectious disease is far from over. So we really do need to keep developing newer and more powerful antibiotics.

There is another time bomb lurking. Because of international travel, diseases once confined to other Third World nations can be easily transmitted to persons in industrialized nations. Another good reason to have antibiotics.

As a medical doctor, I know firsthand how important antibiotics are when it comes to infectious disease. I've been fortunate enough to have witnessed miracles. It seems like almost everyday during the cold and flu season alone, I have patients visit me who are barely able to take their next breath—but when given the proper dosage of these breakthrough healers of the Twentieth Century their illnesses clear up quickly, usually within days.

Working in emergency settings, I've seen antibiotics save lives of children and elderly alike who are afflicted with potentially deadly salmonellosis that may arise from bacterially contaminated food. I've seen penicillin save rural veterinarians from anthrax infection.

And, of course, we always make sure these days that patients receive antibiotics prior to virtually every type of surgery to prevent post-operative infectious complications.

Antibiotics now are used for treatment of ulcers and chronic upper respiratory infections, as well as prostatitis and cystitis.

There is even strong evidence that a course of antibiotics every now and then can reduce the risk of heart disease and arthritis.

There is no doubt: antibiotics are one of the greatest breakthroughs in public health in the history of medicine. There is no question that these miracle agents have saved millions of lives.

So, the Doctor Prescribed Antibiotics... Now What Do You Do?

MAKING ANTIBIOTICS WORK BETTER

And yet for all of their benefits, we doctors also know that antibiotics sometimes pose complications for our patients. What's more, we now know that their efficacy can be positively enhanced through specific nutritional strategies.

Indeed, although usually not life threatening, antibiotics' complications and adverse effects can be minimized and handled quite nicely through such nutritional intervention. This is important, as I have often seen patients who, due to medical necessity, must take antibiotics for a month or longer. Easing any complications such as diarrhea, constipation or impaired immune function is one of the keys to insuring that patients take their medicine for the fully prescribed course of time.

In addition, a large number of antibiotics adversely affect the function of immune-related white blood cells.[1]

✦ Antibiotics may inhibit various types of white blood cells' powers of phagocytosis (the ingestion by a white blood cell of a microorganism, cell particle or other matter).

✦ The reactivity of some types of white blood cells called lymphocytes or B-cells may be impaired. These cells produce protein molecules known as antibodies that, with their uniquely shaped sites, combine with viruses to disable them.

Impaired immune function enables the bacterial pathogens to persist in the body, which, under certain circumstances, may be the basis for chronic infection. Reduced immunity can lead to otherwise unnecessary long-term antibiotic therapy. This may also lead to secondary infections and fungal illnesses.

What's more, almost all antibiotics can cause nausea, vomiting, diarrhea, or, conversely, sometimes constipation, nutrient depletion, and overgrowth of nonsusceptible organisms, including fungi and protozoa, most notably candida (see table, pages 23-25).

Super (or secondary) infections are another possible result of antibiotic treatment. It should be noted that while antibiotics eliminate both friendly and harmful bacteria, there are a number of drug-resistant harmful bacteria that not only survive antibiotics but also thrive. Following antibiotic therapy and the body's depleted levels of friendly bacteria, these newly empowered drug-resistant pathogenic bacteria now have an unobstructed playing field. Among the drug-resistant bacteria are *staphylococcus* and *pseudomonas* species. Worse yet, superinfections may not only be limited to the gastrointestinal tract only but may spread and become systemic.

Given that more and more drug-resistant bacteria are evolving, there is also an increase in prescriptions of highly potent antibiotics. These broad-spectrum, extremely effective antibiotics hit both friend and foe alike, since they are "equal opportunity"

SPECIAL DATA DELIVERY

Almost any antibiotic will change the bacterial balance in the intestines. Solid data suggest that the use of antibiotics before surgery results in decreased levels of both aerobic and anaerobic bacteria to between 20 and 25 percent of their original amounts.[2] While pre-surgical dispensation of antibiotics assuredly and importantly leads to a decline in the rate of post-operative infections, it also induces a massive die-off rate of beneficial bacteria in the intestine.

The enemy of your enemy is my friend

*Antibiotics can annihilate
our colonic friends and get
us into big trouble—fast*

*So, the Doctor
Prescribed
Antibiotics...
Now What
Do You Do?*

CYBER
CHAT
ROOM

What
Other
Doctors
Say...

According to Michael D. Gershon, author of *The Second Brain* (Harper-Collins, 1998), "One reason that the bacteria in the lumen of the colon do not break out and infect the body is that they are at war with one another. No one kind of germ gains ascendancy and takes uncontested possession of colonic turf. The constant competition between otherwise nasty germs helps to keep the bacterial population under control." As Dr. Gershon, who is chairman of the Department of Anatomy and Cell Biology at Columbia University, College of Physicians and Surgeons, points out, "It really is a case of 'the enemy of my enemy is my friend.' Our bacterial companions in the colon may be repulsive, but we still have to take good care of them. Taking an antibiotic, therefore, is not without risk. Killing germs in the colon can be a hazardous venture. Antibiotics that annihilate our colonic friends can get us into big trouble and very fast."

killers. That means that the floral ecology in the intestine is severely perturbed. This ecological vacuum created by the destruction of friendly bacteria is quickly filled by pathogenic microorganisms. With billions of attachment sites open in the intestine, the harmful bacteria have the opportunity to move in and take hold.

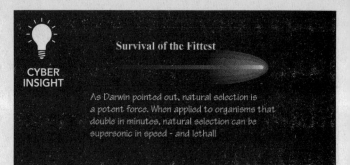

The rapid deployment of the bad bacteria leads to the repopulation of the intestine by numerous disease-causing microorganisms. For example, the overgrowth of *Clostridium difficile*, an especially harmful bacterium, gives rise to a condition called *Pseudomembraneous enterocolitis*. The condition, produced by this opportunistic invader, includes bloody diarrhea, pain, catastrophic weight loss and ulcerations of the intestinal lining.

Many kinds of bacteria are killed by antibiotics, but not all. Those that are not killed are those that are most resistant. As Charles Darwin pointed out, natural selection is a potent force. When applied to organisms that double in minutes, natural selection is not just potent but fast. Selection by antibiotics is thus not a good move for modern medicine. The therapeutic value of drug after drug has been lost as bacteria adapt to them and circumvent their efforts.

Antibiotic resistance is a fact of bacterial life, and it is a difficulty that the indiscriminate use of antibiotics has made far more serious than it used to be, continues Dr. Gershon. Since antibiotics are routinely added to chicken feed and used to address other agricultural problems, the proportion of resistant organisms increases every year. This problem is compounded by the large number of doctors who prescribe antibiotics without first determining whether the disease they wish to treat is due to a susceptible organism. By killing some bacteria and not others, the administration of an antibiotic may eliminate the competition between germs in the colon, so that one strain, which appears to be resistant, achieves dominance. In essence, the drug selects a bug. The resistant strain is thus dangerous for a number of reasons. One is that it has been liberated from the restraint imposed on it by the other bacteria that normally compete with antibiotic-resistant organisms. The point is that the resistant bacteria are hard to eliminate because it is difficult to find a nontoxic drug that can kill them. The resistant organisms, therefore, are likely to cause a rip–roaring florid colitis infection of the colon. They can also escape from the colon and invade the body. Some of the antibiotic-resistant strains of bacteria, such as *Clostridia difficile*, make toxins that peel the lining of the colon right off the organ and lead to an explosive, debilitating and frequently lethal form of diarrhea.

So, the Doctor Prescribed Antibiotics... Now What Do You Do?

Another pathogenic bacterium that can take advantage of the void created by the elimination of friendly bacteria is *Staphylococcus aureus*. Its overgrowth can also result in toxic shock syndrome and it can become very resistant. Known as methicillin-resistant staph or MRSA, this strain requires far more potent vancomycin therapy.

The matter of drug-resistant bacteria is very serious with profound implications. Most recently, for example, the Reuters news service reported that this drug-resistant form of bacteria has been found in rural Native American communities, demonstrating that so-called superbugs are moving out of their hospital breeding grounds and into the community.[3] According to health researchers, the MRSA strain has been found now in Minnesota among Native Americans living in the countryside. That means the infections resisted treatment with methicillin and can be killed only by vancomycin, which is considered a last-ditch antibiotic.

Only a quarter of the patients with MRSA had been in a hospital, a long-term care facility or had any of the other usual risk factors for getting a drug-resistant infection. Such cases of MRSA infection outside the hospital had been seen before only in isolated incidents in Australia, Chicago and Canada.

Scientists say drug-resistant bacteria evolve when they are exposed to antibiotics over time—which most frequently happens in hospitals. Patients who get antibiotics for months on end become breeding grounds for the bacteria, because a few will always survive the antibiotic—and these will be the ones genetically predisposed to resist the drug. The longer these survive, the more they multiply and the resistance spreads.

When the friendly bacteria are decimated by antibiotics, other harmful bacteria, yeast and fungi already living in the body, which were held in strict check by the friendly bacteria, begin to multiply profusely. The overgrowth of one especially potent yeast-like fungus, *Candida albicans*, leads to a potentially serious condition called candidasis or yeast infection. Depending on its locale of action, candidiasis can inflame the tongue, mouth or the rectum. It could also cause vaginitis and may be instrumental in triggering a range of mental and emotional symptoms, including irritability, anxiety and even depression. Many allergies that manifest themselves as digestive disorders, such as bloating, heartburn, constipation and diarrhea also have been causally linked to yeast overgrowth.

Knowing how to use antibiotics in a safe and effective manner is critically important to doctors, pharmacists, and consumers alike. And to children. The American Academy of Pediatrics recently observed that 95 percent of children in the United States will have been treated with antibiotics for a middle ear infection by the age of five.

Sounds pretty ominous. But Dr. Gershon knows of what he speaks. We really do need to care for our friends in our colon.

The key to preventing such a condition from striking you or your loved ones is to replenish the body's population of friendly bacterial organisms.

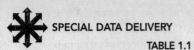

TABLE 1.1

Antibiotic Uses, Complications, Nutrient-related Interactions

Drug	Common Uses	Potential Adverse Health Effects
All antibiotics	To fight off and prevent bacterial infections.	The use of antibiotics is limited because bacteria may evolve resistance to them. The problem of resistance has been increased by the inappropriate use of antibiotics for the treatment of common viral infections. Such use removes antibiotic-sensitive bacteria and allows the development of antibiotic-resistant bacteria. Tuberculosis, for example, once nearly eradicated in the developed countries, is increasing partly because of resistance to antibiotics.
Penicillins	Are used to treat such diseases as syphilis, gonorrhea, meningitis, and anthrax.	Side effects of the penicillins, while rare, can include allergic reactions such as skin rashes fever, and anaphylactic shock.
Cephalosporins	May be used to treat strains of meningitis and in orthopedic, abdominal, and pelvic surgery.	Rare reactions to the cephalosporins include skin rash and anaphylactic shock.

Drug	Common Uses	Potential Adverse Health Effects
Aminoglycosides (e.g., streptomycin)	Inhibit bacterial protein synthesis and are sometimes used in combination with penicillin.	These tend to be more toxic than other antibiotics. Rare adverse effects associated with prolonged use of aminoglycosides include hearing loss and kidney damage.
Macrolides (e.g., erythromycin)	The macrolides work by interrupting protein synthesis. Erythromycin, one of the macrolides, is often used as a substitute for penicillin against streptococcal and pneumococcal infections. Other uses for macrolides include treating diphtheria and bacteremia.	Side effects may include nausea, vomiting, and diarrhea.
Sulfonamides	The sulfonamides are synthetic antibiotics that are effective against many types of bacteria, although some bacteria have developed resistance to them. Sulfonamides are now used only in very specific situations, such as urinary system infection and in lyme disease.	Side effects may include disruption of the gastrointestinal tract and hypersensitivity.

Drug	Nutrients Depleted	More Adverse Reactions
Penicillins, cephalosporins, fluoroquinolones, macrolides, aminoglycosides, sulfonamides	*Lactobacillus acidophilus, Bifidobacteria bifidum* (bifidus); vitamins B_1, B_2, B_3, B_6, B_{12}, K; biotin, inositol	Increased susceptibility to pathogens; constipation; diarrhea.
	Calcium Magnesium Iron	Irregular heartbeat and blood pressure; osteoporosis; tooth decay.
		Asthma, cardiovascular problems, cramps, osteoporosis, premenstrual syndrome.
		Anemia, brittle nails, fatigue, hair loss, weakness.
Tetracyclines, sulfonamides	*Lactobacillus acidophilus, Bifidobacteria bifidum* (bifidus); vitamins B_1, B_2, B_3, B_6, B_{12}, biotin, inositol	Increased susceptibility to pathogens; constipation; diarrhea.
Neomycin	Beta-carotene; vitamins A and B_{12}	Fatigue.
Co-trimoxazole sulfonamides	*Lactobacillus acidophilus, Bifidobacteria bifidum* (bifidus); folic acid	Increased susceptibility to pathogens; constipation; diarrhea.

TWO

Gastrointestinal Ecology Under Attack

ONE AREA OF HEALTH BEING STUDIED most intensively is the body's gastrointestinal (GI) system. This is because of its direct contact with eaten foods and the complexity of its functions regarding nutrient assimilation and healthy immune function. The GI system is the potential target for many functional foods and dietary supplements. It is the gate to systemic health or unhealth.

It is increasingly being recognized that the microbiology of the human GI system can exert a major role in host health, both in a positive and negative manner. One important aspect is the manipulation of the composition of the gut flora towards a potentially more healthy community. As such, attempts have been made to learn how increased numbers of beneficial bacterial species (such as bifidobacte-

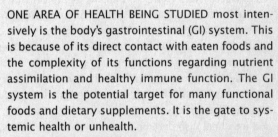

EXTENT OF THE PROBLEM

CYBER
INSIGHT

One third of patients present to their physicians with gastrointestinal problems:

- Constipation & Diarrhea
- Bloating & Flatulence
- Heartburn
- Anal Itching

ria and lactobacilli), both of which may exert various health-promoting properties.

Yet, the antibiotics that your doctor may have prescribed for helping you to get through your cold or flu this winter could end up impairing your body's immunity. That is because—in addition to their deleterious effects on white blood cells—antibiotics have a broad-spectrum anti-bacterial effect *and* frequently destroy populations of both unfriendly and friendly bacteria that are essential to normal immune function.

Your body is composed of 75 trillion cells. Ninety percent of these cells live within the 29 feet which form your intestinal tract. That's right, 90 percent of the cells of your body actually comprise an ecosystem of microorganisms which reside within your guts. This amazing mathematical observation is possible because the size of most microbes is much smaller than human cells.

A healthy population of friendly bacteria in your gastrointestinal tract is critical to your overall health. Indeed, few people realize the enormous impact of pathogenic bacteria, parasites and intestinal disorders on human well-being. Worldwide, diarrheal diseases (bacterial as well as parasitic) constitute the greatest single cause of morbidity and mortality. In the United states, diarrheal diseases caused by intestinal infection are the third leading cause of morbidity and mortality.

Even more prevalent than acute diarrheal illnesses is the occurrence of more subtle intestinal bacterial imbalances which produce a host of common symptoms and result in an obvious lack of wellness. We may know this condition as irritable bowel syndrome, immune dysfunction or simply dyspepsia. But it can mask itself with many different symptoms. Many of these can be traced back to use of antibiotics either during a single complete course of therapy or among persons who seem to be chronically in need of antibiotics. Of growing concern to doctors like myself is the adverse impact that antibiotics can have on gastrointestinal health. The human large intestine, the colon, is the region of the gastrointestinal tract that is most heavily colonized by bacteria. These colonizing bacteria are variously termed flora or microbiota, and estimates are that one gram of the colon may contain as many as 100 billion bacteria. Bacteria often cause a process called fermentation. This is the process by which any group of living organisms such as yeasts, molds and certain bacteria, in the absence of air or oxygen, cause the breakdown of molecules and yield energy. In particular, the colon's bacteria are able to produce a wide range of compounds that have varying effects on gut physiology, some negative, and some with positive health effects, for the entire body. For example, it is thanks to friendly bacteria that our body is able to manufacture and assimilate many essential vitamins and minerals.

Gastrointestinal Ecology Under Attack

Today, medical scientists are actively pursuing work that will allow nutritional manipulation of the contents of gut flora to generate a more healthy bacterial community. The focus is to increase the numbers and activities of those groups of bacteria which have health-promoting activities.

We take our gastrointestinal tract or gut for granted. We really shouldn't. In his book *The Second Brain*, Dr. Gershon dubs that entire gastrointestinal system, the body's second nervous system. He notes, "The brain is not the only place in the body that's full of neurotransmitters. A hundred million neurotransmitters line the length of the gut, approximately the same number that is found in the brain . . . . The brain in the bowel has got to work right or no one will have the luxury to think at all." The gut or the intestine is within the body but it is its own world. In experimental studies, even when all nerves connecting the bowel to the brain and spinal cord were severed, "the law of the intestine" prevailed, and digestion continued. Let's not take gastrointestinal health for granted!

It has been estimated that as many as 50 different families of bacteria reside in the colon, comprising several hundred individual species. The activities of colonic bacteria are affected by a number of different factors. The availability of the food and energy source for the bacteria is one such factor. Also, important are the pH and the availability and distribution of oxygen in the colon. It should be noted that for some bacteria that thrive in the colon, oxygen is lethal. For others, they survive just as well in the absence as in the presence of oxygen. The bacteria that multiply and grow in the absence of oxygen are numerically by far the largest group. These are called *anaerobic* bacteria.

GOOD GUYS, BAD GUYS

Generally speaking, intestinal bacteria can be divided into two broad groups: those that are beneficial and those that are harmful to human beings. Health-promoting effects of beneficial bacteria include stimulation of the immune system, lowering of the gas distention problem, improved digestion/absorption of essential nutrients and synthesis of vitamins. Bifidobacteria and lactobacilli are examples of bacteria that are beneficial. In contrast, pathogenic effects of the harmful bacteria include diarrhea, infections, liver damage, cancer and intestinal putrefaction.

All bacteria, good and bad, are important—much as all animal species are important to an ecological system. Each bacterial species that grows in the colon has a specific ecological niche to fulfill. The composition of bacteria—that is, the relative distribution of the "good" and the "bad" bacteria—in an individual's colon remains fairly stable over long periods of time. As such, there is a finely tuned balance in the colon from which the body derives health benefits and the digestive system works smoothly without causing any ailments or discomfort. However, this balance can be easily disrupted.

ANTIBIOTICS: LETHAL THREAT TO GASTROINTESTINAL ECOLOGY

Perhaps the greatest threat today to our body's bacterial ecology are antibiotics. These modern medical miracles work as efficient "torpedoes" and eliminate invading bacteria. Antibiotics, however, are also "equal opportunity" torpedoes, and kill both the good and the bad bacteria equally effectively.

By the time the antibiotic course is run, people feel drained, exhausted and may have succumbed to antibiotic-associated diarrhea. Children on antibiotics are especially susceptible to antibiotic-associated bacterial influences that cause diarrhea. Diarrhea may resolve itself, which it normally does, particularly in children, but antibiotics frequently perturb the ecological balance in the colon and allow the overgrowth of harmful bacteria. Left to itself, this imbalance could poten- *Gastrointestinal* tially disturb the intestinal "ecosys- *Ecology Under* tem" irrevocably. *Attack*

THE GUTS OF LIFE SPILL

CYBER INSIGHT When a person does not have good gastrointestinal health, the following associated symptoms occur:

- Fluctuations in Weight
- Mood Disturbance
- Concentration Difficulties
- More Systemic Disease

DYSBIOSIS: GASTROINTESTINAL ECOLOGY UNBALANCED

Gastrointestinal imbalance is usually referred to as *dysbiosis*. You know scientists and doctors: we like to use fancy words which leave the average person wondering what the heck we're jabbering about. Well, put simply, dysbiosis is one of those fancy words for a condition that occurs when the population of organisms residing within the gastrointestinal tract becomes unbalanced, often resulting in acute or chronic sickness.

Normally, populations of pathogenic flora are kept in balance by competition from good bacteria and because of *symbiosis*, which is the mutually interdependent relationship among the hundreds of intestinal microbial species. The problem is that after antibiotics have wiped out all or much of the entire gastrointestinal landscape, the bad bacteria have the upper hand, especially because they love the types of foods and simple sugars that we typically consume in our diet, such as refined sugar found in candy, baked goods and soft drinks. So, when the balance of good and bad bacteria is disturbed by antibiotics, it's the bad bacteria that get the head start in repopulating the barren property within your gastrointestinal tract. And especially consider this: the kind of food people who are sick or have been sick love to eat is what we call comfort food: you know, hamburgers, milk shakes, fries—the very kind of food that promotes the growth of disease-causing bacteria.

Dysbiosis results from abnormal fermentation in the small intestine.[4] In the large intestine, some fermentation is desirable because it produces butyrate and other short chain fatty acids that nourish the cells of the intestinal wall.[5] In the small intestine, however, growth of yeast, fungi and/or fermenting bacteria can result in damage to the gut lining, absorption of toxic by-products, and impaired absorption of nutrients.[6]

Repeated use of broad-spectrum antibiotics and steroid medications can set up conditions for opportunistic overgrowth of organisms that are not affected by the drugs or that are able to re-colonize rapidly once treatment has ended. This is particularly true of yeast and fungal organisms. Their metabolic products appearing in urine are the strongest physical evidence of intestinal overgrowth of these organisms. As an internist, I can't tell you how often I have seen patients treated with antibiotics, especially women patients, whose bodies are overrun by candida. For men, such treatment often results in residual urinary tract bacteria, resulting in urinary tract infections and prostatitis which is an inflammation of the prostate gland.

Dysbiosis Poses Many Health Problems

So dysbiosis is a fancy word for the imbalance of bacteria in your gastrointestinal tract. But what we need to keep in mind is that persistent dysbiosis can have serious health consequences.

It surely causes gastrointestinal problems, but it can also lead to a weakened immune system. As the body loses its ability to cope with the offending infections and pathogens, a host of chronic conditions appear that, on the surface, may have precious little to do with gastrointestinal disturbances.

That means gastrointestinal health has far-reaching implications for general health, much more so than is commonly recognized. Indeed, as an internist, I *Gastrointestinal* have often had to do quite a bit of *Ecology Under* medical sleuthing to track down my *Attack* patients' complaints finally to dysbiosis or an imbalance of their gastrointestinal bacteria. But once we do so and then take appropriate pathways to enhance the healing response, my patients respond quite favorably.

The recognition that healthy intestinal flora is essential for good health first developed over one hundred years ago during the birth of the science of microbiology. But widespread recognition by today's generation of medical doctors has been slow in coming.

Fortunately, the importance to human health of the intestinal microflora has been more widely recognized by doctors in recent years. This is probably because ever-increasing environmental challenges (e.g., antibiotics, oral contraceptives, food additives and especially refined sugar) have contributed to the greater prevalence of disharmony in the ecology of the intestines.

I mean, imagine this: we've only had refined sugar for one hundred to two-hundred years. Refined sugar is the favorite chow for disease-causing bacteria. We've only had antibiotics for about fifty years, and they're probably the most efficient weapon ever devised for killing off bacteria, both good and bad. No wonder do many people today are victims of dysbiosis!

So this idea that our body's bacteria balance can be upset is a relatively new concept to medicine. The ancients knew what we're talking about (and if you want to know what the ancient Egyptians knew about enhancing immunity and caring for the gastrointestinal tract, then turn to Chapter 5). But when it comes to modern doctors, be patient. Modern medicine is just catching up to this ancient knowledge and the fact that the consequences of dysbiosis appear to extend beyond immediately obvious gastrointestinal distress; evidence points to the influence of nutrient intake, intestinal permeability, and changes in levels of essential fatty acids as the root cause of a number of systemic disorders. Other studies have implicated intestinal bacterial imbalances as a basis for conditions ranging from recurrent infections and immune breakdown to chronic fatigue. More familiar to many of my patients are conditions such as irritable bowel syndrome, fibromyalgia, leaky gut syn-

SPECIAL DATA DELIVERY

Costly National Concern

Today, we know that digestive diseases and other conditions related to healthy or unhealthy balances of intestinal flora have an enormous impact on our health. They are extremely costly in all ways.

Digestive diseases, which often are caused in part by, or result in, dysbiosis, cost nearly $107 billion in direct health care expenditures in 1992.7 Digestive diseases result in nearly 200 million sick days, 50 million visits to physicians, 16.9 million days lost from school, 10 million hospitalizations, and nearly 200,000 deaths per year.

The most costly digestive diseases are gastrointestinal disorders such as diarrheal infections ($4.7 billion); gallbladder disease ($4.5 billion); colorectal cancer ($4.5 billion); liver disease ($3.2 billion); and peptic ulcer disease ($2.5 billion).

Cancers of the digestive tract, which includes the colon, the gallbladder, and the stomach, are responsible for 117,000 deaths yearly. Noncancerous digestive diseases cause 74,000

drome, wasting syndrome, diverticulitis, hemorrhoids, and can-cer—all of which may have their genesis in an upset in the gastrointestinal tract's bacterial population.

FAR-REACHING HEALTH CONSEQUENCES

Not surprisingly, dysbiosis or dysbacteriosis and its prevention or treatment are among the most topical and challenging problems we doctors face today.[8]

In dysbiosis—when protective friendly bacterial species are reduced in population—even organisms traditionally thought to have little ability to cause disease, including usually benign bacteria, yeasts, and some parasites, can

Gastrointestinal Ecology Under Attack

SPECIAL
DATA
DELIVERY
continued

deaths a year, with 36 percent caused by chronic liver disease and cirrhosis.

Of the 440 million acute noncancerous medical conditions reported in the United States annually, more than 22 million are for acute digestive conditions, with 11 million from gastroenteritis and 6 million from indigestion, nausea, and vomiting.

Digestive diseases have an enormous impact on health and the health-care system in the United States. New technologies and new drugs have revolutionized the understanding and treatment of peptic ulcer disease and gastrointestinal esophageal reflux disease (GERD). Successful outcomes of future research will hopefully continue to reduce the economic and health care costs related to diagnosing and treating digestive diseases. But the bottom line remains: your body desperately requires healthy intestinal flora, while many environmental and dietary conditions threaten this balance.

induce illness by altering our nutritional status or immune response. In today's world, where we're looking to maximize our health, having suboptimal nutritional status or immune response may leave us predisposed to a host of common ailments including diarrhea, constipation, irritable bowel syndrome, colon cancer, allergies, vaginitis, increased susceptibility to infection, food cravings, lack of mental clarity, chronic fatigue, fibromyalgia, hypoglycemia symptoms and many more symptoms that may be indirectly or directly related to poor nutrient assimilation and bacterial imbalances.

Dysbiosis can produce obvious intestinal symptoms of diarrhea, burning, bloating, cramping and constipation. Equally important, however, are the effects on tissues far from the intestinal site, such as the brain, joints and muscles, as well as on the immune system. Effects can be as diverse as headaches, learning disorders, insomnia, immune dysfunction, behavioral disorders, chronic fatigue, joint pain, and nutritional deficiencies.

Dysbiosis can be a significant factor in many health problems. Abnormal gut fermentation has adverse effects on B vitamins, zinc and magnesium.[9] These nutritional deficits help to explain how unhealthy gut fermentation may cause significant, yet unrelated adverse effects on health.

In our quest for optimal physical and emotional health and longevity, having a healthy intestine is of critical importance. For longevity and to assure optimal protection from age-related illness, having a healthy colon is of immeasurable importance.

CYBER INSIGHT

How Do You Know if You Have Dysbiosis?

The most common symptoms of intestinal dysbiosis are bloating, abdominal cramping, and diarrhea. In other words, indigestion is a surefire sign of dysbiosis. Lactose intolerance, increased gut permeability, food intolerances, fatigue and immune suppression frequently accompany intestinal dysbiosis.

MOST COMMON CONDITIONS ASSOCIATED WITH DYSBIOSIS (BACTERIAL IMBALANCES)

Let's look at some of the most common major diseases associated with imbalances of friendly bacteria. We will present additional information on healing many of these conditions in later chapters.

Inflammatory Bowel Disease

Inflammatory bowel disease is a term describing an intestinal condition characterized by a combination of abdominal pain; constipation; diarrhea; increased secretion of colon-related mucus; and

Gastrointestinal Ecology Under Attack

CYBER INSIGHT

Common Symptoms of Intestinal Imbalances

+ Fatigue
+ Flatulence
+ Itchy anus
+ Poor complexion
+ Fatigue after eating
+ Distention/bloating
+ Inability to lose weight
+ Constipation or diarrhea
+ Irritable bowel syndrome
+ Abdominal pain or cramps
+ Irregular bowel movements
+ Rheumatoid arthritis
+ Colon cancer
+ Poor digestion
+ Food allergy
+ Spastic colon
+ Tiredness after meals
+ Hypoglycemia
+ Leaky gut syndrome

CYBER INSIGHT

Major Causes of Dysbiosis

+ Intestinal infection
+ Poor diet—excessive sugar, fat or animal protein
+ Stress—including long-term emotional stress
+ Decreased immune function
+ Decreased intestinal motility (constipation)
+ Drugs—especially antibiotics, oral contraception and cortisone
+ Maldigestion and malabsorption-like substances

dyspeptic symptoms such as flatulence, nausea, anorexia and varying degrees of anxiety or depression.

Inflammatory bowel disease refers to two chronic intestinal disorders: Crohn's disease and ulcerative colitis. This condition affects between two to six percent of Americans or an estimated 300,000 to 500,000 people. The causes of Crohn's disease and ulcerative colitis are not yet known, but a leading theory suggests that some agent, perhaps a virus or bacterium, alters the body's immune response, triggering an inflammatory reaction in the intestinal wall. Many health professionals believe that this virus or bacterium is most likely to exert its disease-causing effect when the body's balance of friendly bacteria is upset.

The onset for both diseases peaks during young adulthood. An individual with either disease may suffer persistent abdominal pain, bowel sores, diarrhea, fever, intestinal bleeding, or weight loss.

If your doctor thinks you have either Crohn's disease or ulcerative colitis, a variety of procedures and tests such as endoscopy and barium GI studies are available to confirm disease. Once diagnosed, treatment options may include medications, dietary changes, and sometimes surgery to remove the diseased bowel. Remission and cure is possible in either condition, but both conditions may persist over an individual's lifetime. Restoration of the balance of friendly bacteria to the gastrointestinal tract often helps and is essential to recovery.

 Cyber Disease Description—CROHN'S DISEASE. Crohn's disease primarily involves the small bowel and the proximal colon. It may cause the intestinal wall to thicken and cause narrowing of the bowel channel, possibly blocking the intestinal tract. The result is abnormal membrane function, including nutrient malabsorption.

About 90 percent of patients with Crohn's disease experience frequent and progressive symptoms of abdominal pain, diarrhea, and weight loss. This can lead to extreme weight loss seen in other wasting conditions such as cancer and AIDS.

The most commonly used drugs to treat Crohn's are sulfasalazine, prednisolone, mesalamine, metronidazole, and azathioprine.

If a patient does not respond to oral medications, the doctor may recommend surgery. Although surgery relieves chronic symptoms, Crohn's disease often recurs at the location where the healthy parts of the bowel were rejoined. The length of time that a Crohn's patient is in remission is not predictable. Again, rebalancing the body's bacterial populations can help.

Gastrointestinal Ecology Under Attack

A recent case report from my own clinical practice provides an excellent example of the healing powers of inulin.

A True Life Inulin-Healing Story from the Internet M.D.

Kathy, aged 46, had wasting syndrome with longstanding Crohn's disease and multiple gastrointestinal problems, including diarrhea and inability to gain weight. In fact, Kathy had been on medical marijuana (Marinol—the pill) for the last six months just so that she could eat enough to maintain her thin frame of 96 pounds.

When we put Kathy on inulin, a miracle was hoped for but not expected. For her, it was one more thing that she really didn't want to take, but she was convinced that along with prayer, good things might happen. No promises were made.

However, amazingly, within forty-eight hours, she noticed that her belching and nausea were improved. Her intake of Lomotil (usually six a day) dropped 33 percent. Her bowel movements became firmer and regular. The most important thing she noticed was that she was beginning to feel healthy again.

Cyber Disease Description—ULCERATIVE COLITIS. Ulcerative colitis (UC) is an inflammatory disorder affecting the inner lining of the large intestine. The inflammation originates in the lower colon and spreads through the entire colon. Blood in the stool is the most common and distinct symptom of ulcerative colitis. As with Crohn's disease, doctors diagnose ulcerative colitis by conducting a complete physical exam and other procedures such as barium enema, endoscopy and intestinal biopsy.

Patients with mild or severe ulcerative colitis are initially treated with sulfasalazine. Steroids are usually added in high doses. Other experimental drugs to treat ulcerative colitis include budesonide, tixocortol pivalate enema, and beclomethasone dipropionate enema.

Despite new therapies, an estimated 20 to 25 percent of ulcerative colitis patients will need surgery. Surgery cures ulcerative colitis and most patients can go on to lead normal lives—except they may do so with a colostomy bag. I think it is so important that we first try natural healing pathways first.

Cyber Disease Description—
Irritable Bowel Syndrome

Irritable bowel syndrome (IBS) is a common functional disorder of the intestines estimated to affect five million Americans. The cause of IBS is not yet known. Doctors refer to IBS as a functional disorder because there is no sign of disease when the colon is examined. But functional, in this case, means "dysfunctional."

Doctors believe that people with IBS experience abnormal patterns of colonic movement and absorption capabilities. The IBS colon is highly sensitive, overreacting to any stimuli such as gas, stress, or eating high-fat or fiber-rich foods.

Patients with IBS often experience alternating bouts of constipation and diarrhea. Although abdominal pain and cramps are among the most common IBS symptoms, pain or discomfort alone is not sufficient to make the diagnosis. However, when a bowel movement or the passage of gas temporarily relieves pain and cramps, a doctor may suspect IBS and begin therapy.

IBS is frequently diagnosed after doctors exclude more serious intestinal diseases through a detailed medical history and complete physical examination.

There is no standard way of treating IBS, but multiple drugs are often used. Of critical importance is restoration of friendly bacteria to the gut and appropriate lifestyle and dietary changes. In addition, antidepressants and psychotherapy are frequently part of the program.

Gastrointestinal Ecology Under Attack

 Cyber Disease Description—
Peptic Ulcer

Peptic ulcer disease, estimated to affect 4.5 million people in the United States, is a chronic inflammation of the stomach and duodenum. Peptic ulcer is responsible for substantial human suffering and a large economic burden. Every year four million people report missing approximately six days from work because of their ulcers.

Peptic ulcers result from the breakdown of the lining of the stomach and duodenum caused by increased stomach acid and pepsin and *Helicobacter pylori (H. pylori)*. One type of ulcer occurs in the stomach, the other in the duodenum, the first part of the small intestine. Duodenal ulcers are much more common than stomach ulcers, which have a greater risk of malignancy.

There are no specific symptoms of gastric and duodenal ulcers. However, upper abdominal pain and nausea are the most common symptoms of peptic ulcer disease. Ulcer pains usually occur an hour or two after meals, or in the early morning hours and abate after food or antacids have been eaten. Definitive diagnosis of peptic ulcer disease requires endoscopy, which also allows a doctor to obtain biopsy samples, if needed. The Food and Drug Administration's 1996 approval of a safe, effective breath test makes noninvasive diagnosis of ulcers possible.

In the 1950s, doctors thought stress and diet caused peptic ulcer disease. Treatment during those years concentrated on bed rest, bland foods, and in some cases, hospitalization.

But in 1982, the *Helicobacter pylori* bacterium was isolated from gastric biopsies of patients with chronic gastritis, and is now believed to be the major cause of peptic ulcer disease. *H. pylori* is found in almost 100 percent of patients with duodenal ulcers and in 80 percent of patients with gastric ulcers.

Recently, an independent panel of medical experts convened by the National Institutes of Health confirmed that using a combination of antimicrobial drugs for at least two weeks will eradicate *H. pylori* in a majority of patients, thus reducing the relapse rate of ulcers. A combination of Pepto-Bismol, tetracycline, and metronidazole effectively kills *H. pylori* in approximately 90 percent of patients. The FDA recently approved a two-drug combination of clarithromycin (Biaxin) and omeprazole (Prilosec) to cure stomach ulcers and prevent them from coming back.

As a clinician, I have found that rebuilding the body's population of beneficial bacteria is very helpful.

Cyber Disease Description—
Infant Constipation
Chronic functional constipation is common in infants, especially in bottle-fed babies who may be lacking viable populations of friendly bifidus bacteria. Researchers from the Department of Pediatrics, Ospedale Civile Maggiore, University of Verona, Italy, investigated the composition of the intestinal ecosystem in chronic functional constipation.[10] These researchers discovered that constipated children presented a significant increase in clostridia and bifidobacteria in feces compared to healthy subjects. Different species of clostridia and enterobacteriaceae were also frequently isolated. These intestinal disturbances were linked to dysbiosis, i.e. an imbalance of intestinal bacterial species.

Clearly, maintenance of bacterial balance in the intestinal tract is critical for intestinal health. Dietary changes and food supplements are essential and used frequently to restore beneficial bacteria, normalize digestive function and repair the gut. A high fiber, low sugar diet and increased water intake are also vitally important to maintain healthy intestinal ecology.

However, many people will greatly benefit by positioning inulin on their side. It is a powerful gastrointestinal health enhancer.

Inulin?! What's inulin?

Well, that's what the next part of this book is about.

Gastrointestinal Ecology Under Attack

Are you ready to walk through the door? I can guide you and hold your hand—but I can't do it for you. The next step is yours!

THREE

Inulin—A Good-for-You Functional Food to Enhance Health & Assure Antibiotic Efficacy & Safety

INULIN IS PRECISELY THE PLANT FIBER that will allow your body to use its own healing potential to the fullest. Inulin is the soluble fiber isolated from Jerusalem artichoke—a healthy food from ancient biblical times.

The most important property of inulin is that it acts as a *prebiotic*. That is, it stimulates the multiplication of beneficial bacteria in the colon. The key to our overall health lies in the colon, which is inhabited by billions of bacteria. Some of these bacteria are beneficial to the human health whereas others are harmful. Thus, there is a balance between the "good" and the "bad" bacteria in the colon. Whenever this balance is disturbed, intestinal health suf-

Inulin: A Natural Prebiotic

CYBER INSIGHT

A nondigestible food that enhances health by selectively stimulating the growth and activity of the good bacteria in the colon: *lactobacillus* and *bifidobacteria*

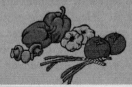

fers. Unless this balance is restored, you will become susceptible to various ailments and infections, because your immune system is not getting the requisite support that it needs when the "good" bacteria are in the right amount. This problem can be especially exacerbated if you take antibiotics in case of an infection. Antibiotics destroy both the good and the bad bacteria in the intestine indiscriminately. That means that the imbalance in the intestinal flora is aggravated.

Nutritional supplementation with Jerusalem artichoke-derived inulin will not only make you feel better but you may also soon forget what it was like to wake up every morning with nausea or to feel tired and "grungy" throughout the day. The goal of this book is to help you minimize your dependence on drugs and maximize your control over your health. Prebiotics are a new way to think about intestinal health. What is more, prebiotics are good for your intestinal health, but they are also good for your blood sugar and good for your cholesterol count. By any standard, prebiotics will change the way we think about both our intestinal and overall health.

Imagine being able to indulge your sweet tooth with real sugar—not a substitute—at one-tenth the usual calories. Imagine a simple, safe pill or powder that can reduce the most common side effects of your doctor's antibiotics, such as gastrointestinal upset, nausea, diarrhea, and constipation.

As a bonus, you would also be guarding against high cholesterol and cancer and promoting better digestion. Your risk for many different types of acute and chronic infectious disease would be reduced dramatically.

As doctors and health scientists explore, with increasing depth and intensity, the relationship between nature's pharmacy and health, functional food science opens new perspectives in nutrition and preventive medicine. Doctors' and scientists' systematic investigation of the interactions between food components or food ingredients and genetic, biochemical, cellular, or physiological functions is a unique way to improve both our knowledge and the role of nutrition in maintaining good health and in preventing disease.

It is thought that the better we understand the mechanism of interactions between food components and specific human biological functions, the more we will be able to demonstrate functional effects for nature's pharmacy—and the easier it will be to accumulate convincing evidence in favor of health promotion and disease prevention.

This may surprise you. But the next trend at the health food store or pharmacy that is already occurring is the sale and consumption of dietary supplements that feed the bacteria in your body that fight diarrhea and other illnesses. Indeed, as Christine Gorman, of *Time* magazine, notes, "Say the word bacteria, and most folks conjure up images of a nasty germ like staphylococcus or salmonella that can make you really sick. But most bacteria aren't bad for you. In fact, consuming extra amounts of some bacteria can actually promote good health. . . . So far, the best results have been seen in the treatment of diarrhea, particularly in children. But researchers are also looking into the possibility that beneficial bacteria may thwart vaginal infections in women, prevent some food allergies in children and lessen symptoms of Crohn's disease, a relatively rare but painful gastrointestinal disorder.

Inulin—A Good-for-You Functional Food to Enhance Health & Assure Antibiotic Efficacy & Safety

"So where have these good germs been lurking all your life? In your intestines, especially the lower section called the colon, which harbors at least 400 species of bacteria. Which ones you have depends largely on your environment and diet. An abundance of good bacteria in the colon generally crowds out stray bad bacteria in your food. But if the bad outnumber the good—for example, after antibiotic treatment for a sinus or an ear infection, which kills normal intestinal germs as well—the result can be diarrhea."[11]

In this regard and for other reasons, enhancing the GI system's population of friendly bacteria represents an exciting therapeutic advance.[12]

PREBIOTICS: A NEW APPROACH TO GREAT HEALTH

A newly developed approach to insuring a healthy flourishing population of friendly bacteria in the gastrointestinal tract is the use of prebiotics, which are added to the diet as feed supplements, much like fertilizer is added to gardens and food crops. Prebiotics are non-digestible food ingredients that may beneficially affect human health by selectively stimulating the growth and/or activity of one or a limited number of beneficial bacterial species already residing in the colon, thus improving the body's overall health and vitality. Increased intake of prebiotics can favorably modulate the colonies of the colon and entire GI system's bacterial population by selectively increasing numbers of specific beneficial strains.[13]

INULIN: PREMIERE PREBIOTIC

Prebiotics represent a nutritional microbial supplement that positively affects health by enhancing the body's microbial balance. Inulin is one of the premiere prebiotics available today.

Inulin is a natural, highly purified fiber taken from the root of the ancient and esteemed biblical food known as Jerusalem artichoke. Inulin is already widely used as a healthy sugar substitute in Europe. Diabetics are well aware of its benefits for normalizing blood sugar levels and its safety—this, in large part, thanks to the pioneering efforts of the former East German government, which recognized both its benign effect on the body's glycemic level and the fact that the Jerusalem artichoke was able to be grown without the high cost of intensive pesticide use.

Inulin is the ultimate *pre*biotic. This non-digestible, medium-chained complex sugar stays intact in the gut, helping to establish the proper balance of beneficial intestinal flora. It is not absorbed but used perhaps like a salt lick to feed the "cattle"—in this case, our gastrointestinal tract's bacteria.

Inulin belongs to a group of naturally occurring complex sugars and carbohydrates containing non-digestible fructooligosaccharides, commonly referred to as FOS in the nutrition industry. Inulin is found in over 36,000 plants worldwide. It has been estimated that as much as one-third of the total vegetation on earth consists of plants that contain inulin. However, the most common inulin-containing plant species include chicory root, asparagus, onions, garlic, barley, and Jerusalem artichoke.

Among these inulin-producing plants, Jerusalem artichoke produces the highest amount of inulofructosaccharides in its tubers, which have been long consumed by the nomads of the Middle East, North American natives, and more recently by Europeans.

Inulin—A Good-for-You Functional Food to Enhance Health & Assure Antibiotic Efficacy & Safety

Sources of Inulin

CYBER INSIGHT

Many vegetables have inulin as part of their fructooligosaccharide composition, but the plant that seems to have the highest content is

Jerusalem Artichoke

It is an oversimplification to consider inulin a complex carbohydrate similar in nature to starch (as found in potatoes) or to simply call it a sugar even though it looks a little like brown sugar and is sweet tasting. The natural flora of the human mouth or intestine does not possess the enzymes required to hydrolyze or digest inulin in the saliva, stomach or intestines. Based on the definition that fibers are polysaccharides impervious to being broken down by enzymes of the digestive system, inulin is more accurately considered a tight, highly woven fiber. Specifically, it is a water-soluble fiber that is large enough to stay intact in the colon, attracting the right kind of bacteria to the "lick."

Because inulin is not digested by the human digestive system, it is extremely calorie spare.*

Although we cannot readily digest inulin, beneficial bacteria that reside in our gut readily use this fiber as a food source. Thus, inulin is a potent growth factor for a number of bacteria and appears to be selectively used by beneficial intestinal bacteria, particularly bifidobacteria. Conversely, unfavorable bacteria such as *Clostridium perfringens* and others are unable to use inulin as a food source. Instead, the bad bacteria go after broken down scraps of refined sugars, which we need to keep out of our system as much as possible.

Inulin is a prebiotic supplement that will be increasingly important for adults, children and infants to use while taking antibiotics, especially in cases of constipation, diarrhea or if they are susceptible to chronic infections. It will also become increasingly important for anyone desiring optimal health because of its beneficial effects on overall gastrointestinal health and energy.

Inulin - A European Delight

CYBER INSIGHT

Inulin is extremely popular in Europe and Japan where you will find it in everything from breakfast cereals to yogurts and chocolate mousses

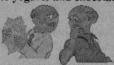

Despite its functional and nutritional benefits, only a few products in the United States at this time contain inulin. "Inulin is still new in this country," says one expert while adding, "inulin is extremely popular in

---

However, due to some fermentation in the large intestine, inulin contributes about 1.5 to 1.6 kilocalories per gram (kcal/gm) to any food product to which it is added.

Europe and Japan. There you see it in everything from breakfast cereals to yogurts and mousses."[14] Other applications include salad dressings, baked goods, low-fat cheeses, no-fat icings and glazes, chocolate, confectionery, surimi, chicken breast, sausages and other processed meats. Even more recently, a low-fat margarine with inulin gel has been developed. In meat products, inulin gel binds water, adds freeze-thaw stability, emulsifies, and adds creaminess.

Inulin—A Good-for-You Functional Food to Enhance Health & Assure Antibiotic Efficacy & Safety

Inulin also has extensive documented historical human use through the consumption of inulin-rich edible plants and fruits. The Aztecs consumed inulin via the dahlia plant. South American Indian cultures consumed artichokes, which are rich sources of inulin; in fact, for millennia, native peoples of Central and South America consumed 50 to 100 grams per day. The Japanese have historically consumed inulin-rich foods such as the yacon plant. Australian aborigines of the nineteenth century consumed a whopping 200 to 300 grams of inulin per day with the murnong plant. In sixteenth century Western Europe, people consumed 35 grams per day through Jerusalem artichokes, Belgian endive (chicory greens), roasted chicory roots, and as a coffee substitute. Today, however, the average daily intake of inulin in the American diet is only about 2.6 grams, which is too bad, since we are missing out on a true health-promoting miracle of nature.[15]

Meanwhile, because inulin has been shown to stimulate growth of bifidobacteria, it has been commercialized in Japan where it is used as a natural medicine to reduce constipation, blood pressure, blood lipids and cholesterol in humans.

Yet, because inulin is sweet, palatable and low in calories, its popularity will, without doubt, continue to rise.

INULIN HEALTH BENEFITS

One of the most dangerous toxic waste sites you will ever encounter is in your own colon. By the time a person is fifty, the colon has accumulated more than 11 pounds of toxic waste! These toxins lead to conditions such as putrefaction, constipation, cancer, and immune dysfunction—but, fortunately, inulin can help us to do something about this condition, especially if populations of beneficial bacteria have been harmed by chronic use of antibiotics.

As a result of disease and its treatment with antibiotics, poor health or poor dietary habits that result in lowered populations of beneficial bacteria, the lining of the intestine may become coated with a leather-like substance of undigested food that serves to nurture unhealthy strains of bacteria and fungi. This process is referred to as putrefaction. In its most advanced form, this condition is known as *Pseudomembraneous colitis*, a not so rare, severe illness in the small and large intestines. Adults, over the age of 60, are mostly affected. It is caused by bacterial infection, usually clostridium, which produces a toxin that triggers the disease. Staphylococcus may also cause the same symptoms: watery diarrhea with occasional abdominal cramps; fever, nausea and vomiting; drop in blood pressure with weak pulse and rapid heartbeat; and disorientation. The name of the disease derives from the presence of characteristic discrete yellow plaques, or pseudomembranes. These plaques are scattered over the entire length of colonic mucosa.

Inulin stimulates viable cultures of acidophilus and bifidobacteria, which have the ability to burrow behind the putrefaction plastered to the intestinal tract and dislodge harmful bacteria and fungi. This is an important first step in detoxifying the colon, especially the small intestine, where most food digestion occurs. This is a mixed neighborhood where both good guy and bad guy bacterial strains (such as *Lactobacillus acidophilus* to *Streptococci*) reside. Unfortunately, it seems that most of the friendly bacteria including lactobacilli and bifidus are quite temporary. Their populations must be nurtured when stress occurs from poor health, poor diet, and use of antibiotics.

This is critical. "When *L. acidophilus* bacteria are present in sufficient numbers, they prevent invading pathogens and opportunistic organisms from finding 'parking spaces' along the walls of the intestine, where nutrients cross into the bloodstream," says medical anthropologist John Heinerman, Ph.D.[16] "If too many harmful bacteria manage to set up colonies, nutrient absorption can be blocked. Fortunately though, when the walls are crowded with acidophilus colonizers, there is no room for newcomers and no way for opportunistic microorganisms to exceed their boundaries. A very desirable characteristic of *L. acidophilus* super strains is that they adhere naturally to the walls of your intestines. These strains, known as *sticker strains*, are the most desirable because they hang onto their parking spaces with great tenacity—without harming the intestinal wall. Most pathogens, like disease-carrying *E. coli*, literally bore holes in the intestinal wall, inducing numerous micro-infections."

Inulin—A Good-for-You Functional Food to Enhance Health & Assure Antibiotic Efficacy & Safety

However, once the small intestine is colonized by a healthy population of beneficial bacteria, "things begin to happen very quickly," notes Dr. Heinerman. "The 'nasties' are compelled to either vacate their premises or else are held in check by the more muscular *L. acidophilus* bacteria."

The most well known effect of inulin is selective stimulation of the growth of bifidobacteria, thus modifying significantly the composition of the colonic microbiota. Such a modification, which has clearly been demonstrated in human volunteers, is meant to be beneficial in part because it is accompanied by a significant reduction in the number of bacteria reported to have disease-causing potential.[17]

Within the framework of research and development of "functional foods," such an effect justifies a "functional claim" for inulin, namely "bifidogenesis" or the creation of hardy, populous colonies of friendly bacteria.

Besides its bifidogenic effect, inulin has additional nutritional properties on digestive physiological parameters like beneficially influencing colonic pH and stool bulking. When people put supplemental inulin into their diet, their constipation is alleviated and frequency and volume of defecation is increased. Besides modulation of GI transit time and fecal bulking, researchers have also noted improvements in glucose absorption with lower blood sugar levels, acidification of colonic content, control of cholesterol bioavailability, reducing serum triglycerides, and lowering blood pressure. Thus, it is well-known that increasing the growth and numbers of beneficial bacteria such as bifidobacteria and lactobacillus has benefits that range from relieving constipation and diarrhea to helping modulate sugar and fat metabolism.

Moreover, it has been shown that inulin, through bifidobacteria fermentation, reduces colonic pH, thereby increasing solubility for various mineral salts. Not surprisingly, it has also been reported that inulin improves the bioavailability of essential minerals such as calcium and magnesium.

SPECIAL DATA DELIVERY

Summary of Inulin Benefits

Inulin offers the following benefits to human gastrointestinal ecology:

- ✦ Stimulates growth of acidophilus, bifidus and faecium.
- ✦ Normalizes fecal pH.
- ✦ Enhances elimination of toxic metabolites.
- ✦ Reduces serum cholesterol and triglyceride levels.
- ✦ Reduces blood pressure among the elderly with high blood lipids.
- ✦ Reduces carbohydrate absorption, thereby normalizing blood glucose.
- ✦ Offers alternative sweeteners for diabetics and dieters.

Through its stimulation of bifidobacteria and suppression of pathogenic bacteria, inulin reduces liver toxins, carcinogens, food intolerances, and provides immune stimulation properties. It also helps to protect against many infectious states including irritable bowel syndrome, and many other bacterially related illnesses.

CYBER INFO SITE

Inulin FAQs

What is inulin?

Inulin is a naturally occurring complex sugar molecule found in Jerusalem artichoke, chicory and other plants with beneficial effects as a food ingredient. It is newly available as a dietary supplement. Inulin is considered to be a health-enhancing food ingredient. Inulin is also known as a prebiotic—since it promotes growth of beneficial bacteria such as acidophilus, bifidus and faecium. Inulin is among the most powerful and beneficial prebiotics known at this time.

Inulin—A Good-for-You Functional Food to Enhance Health & Assure Antibiotic Efficacy & Safety

What are natural sources of inulin?

Inulin is available in a wide variety of edible plants such as banana, garlic, honey, barley, onion, wheat, tomato, and rye. However, most inulin sold today is derived with solvents from chicory. In contrast, inulin derived from the Jerusalem artichoke is naturally extracted and has greater beneficial biological activity. In fact, unpublished industry studies conclusively prove that inulin derived from Jerusalem artichoke possesses greater biological activity.

What about the safety and toxicity of inulin?

Inulin is nontoxic and free of side effects.

Such effects demonstrate interactions between inulin and key functions in the body. And all of these effects are of intense scientific interest.

Until recently, only a limited number of these effects have been investigated, but inulin's amazing health benefits justify many such functional claims, especially as they relate to nutrient assimilation, enhanced resistance to illness, and enhanced antibiotic efficacy and safety. Inulin is just that—a highly efficacious functional food.

FOUR

Inulin & Antibiotics

WE DOCTORS HAVE TO REMEMBER that taking a course of antibiotics can be very difficult on some people, particularly children, the chemically sensitive, and elderly—and anyone with a sensitive stomach. What's more, many people must take antibiotics for protracted periods of time. In one recent case in which I was involved, we had a patient with chronic prostatitis and we had to put him on Levaquin at 250 milligrams (mg) daily for a *month*. Other conditions where prolonged antibiotic use is the rule and not the exception include osteomyelitis, abscesses of the brain, liver or lung, diverticulitis, chronic urinary tract infections, and infections of the heart.

Stomach upset, diarrhea, nausea, constipation, yeast infection, recurrent infections and reduced immune function. These are just a few of the complaints caused by antibiotics. Believe me, when my patients have to take antibiotics for a month or longer or when they are constantly being prescribed them, it's no fun. Yet, in almost all cases, concurrent use of inulin with antibiotics, that is, taking both simultaneously, and continuing to take inulin following use of antibiotics, can play a remarkably beneficial role in reducing side effects and complications.

That's why I am so grateful to nature's pharmacy and the emergence of the powerful healer and antibiotic enhancer, inulin.

Almost all diarrhea caused by antibiotics is a result of the disturbance of the balance of friendly bacteria in the GI sys-

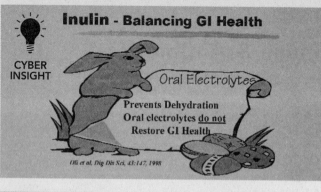

Inulin - Balancing GI Health

CYBER INSIGHT

Oral Electrolytes

**Prevents Dehydration
Oral electrolytes do not
Restore GI Health**

Oli et al, Dig Dis Sci, 43:147, 1998

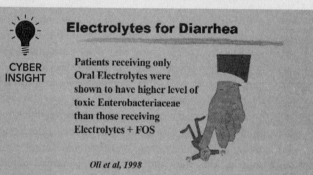

Electrolytes for Diarrhea

CYBER INSIGHT

Patients receiving only
Oral Electrolytes were
shown to have higher level of
toxic Enterobacteriaceae
than those receiving
Electrolytes + FOS

Oli et al, 1998

tem. This is shown clearly in a study from the Department of Biological Sciences, Mississippi State University, Mississippi. There, researchers evaluated the efficacy of an oral electrolyte solution with and without fructooligosaccharides (FOS) for treatment of acute diarrhea induced by cholera toxin.[18] Although total bacterial counts recovered within 24 hours regardless of treatment, densities of potentially toxic *Enterobacteriaceae* were higher for the oral electrolyte solution formula-only treatment. Those receiving the oral electrolyte solution with FOS had more lactobacilli. "Our results show that secretory diarrhea disturbs the normal densities and relative species abundance of the microbiota . . . and that adding FOS to [oral electrolyte solution formulas] accelerates the recovery of bacteria perceived as beneficial while potentially slowing the recovery of pathogenic forms."

This is because when friendly bacterial levels are low due to use of antibiotics, inulin promotes, stabilizes and selectively enhances proliferation of beneficial bacteria into the hostile gastrointestinal environment. In other words, inulin rejuvenates decimated and dying populations of friendly bacteria that have been reduced with antibiotic use. This is critical, for we know with healthy bacterial populations, intestinal upsets such as diarrhea can be avoided or vanquished. We even know that the rotavirus, perhaps the most well known cause of childhood diarrhea in the world, can be overcome with healthy bacterial populations. We think what happens in both children and adults is that once healthy bacterial populations are re-established, they ignite the immune system to recognize this villain and thereby destroy its presence. Or else they simply crowd out the bad guys.

Inulin & Antibiotics

Does inulin really work to re-establish healthy populations of friendly bacteria? *Absolutely!*

Scientific research tells us that feeding inulin to healthy volunteers results in a marked eightfold increase of bifidobacteria with a significant reduction in harmful bacterial strains

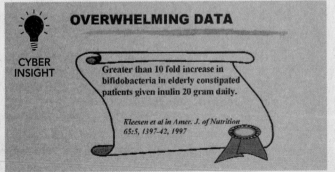

OVERWHELMING DATA

CYBER
INSIGHT

Greater than 10 fold increase in bifidobacteria in elderly constipated patients given inulin 20 gram daily.

Kleesen et al in Amer. J. of Nutrition 65:5, 1397-42, 1997

such as bacteroides, fusobacteria and clostridia.[19] Meanwhile, elderly volunteers given 20 or 40 grams daily of inulin experienced highly significant increases in bifidobacterial counts in feces from $10^{7.9}$ to $10^{8.8}$ and $10^{9.2}$, respectively.[20] That, folks, is a greater than ten-fold increase in friendly bifidobacterial populations.

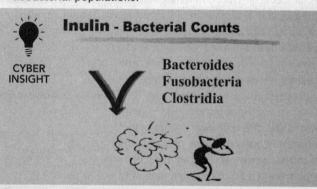

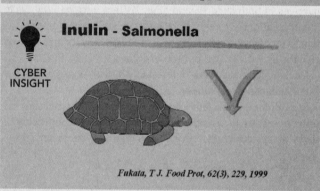

Fukata, T J. Food Prot, 62(3), 229, 1999

By stimulating healthy populations of beneficial bacteria in your gastrointestinal tract, populations of pathogenic bacteria including *Escherichia coli*, *Clostridium perfringers* and others are displaced. Conversely, pathogenic bacteria have been shown to be unable to utilize inulin. Think of inulin as the sheriff in an old wild west town. He'll drive out the bad guys.

The inhibitory effects of inulin on disease-causing bacterial populations have been shown in veterinary studies where smart vets use inulin in place of antibiotics. By the way, this is becoming common practice now in Europe. For example, European regulations now prohibit the use of subtherapeutic dosages of antibiotics in raising poultry. No problem. Now, progressive poultry ranchers use inulin. That's because we know that when chicks are given inulin they gain weight very rapidly. Without inulin, the chicks become infested with disease-causing bacteria such as salmonella. That's bad news all the way around: for consumers, the animals themselves, and the ranchers' bottom lines. These ravenous disease-causing bacteria eat up all the nutrients fed the chicks, causing farmers to use more feed with less weight gain. On the other hand, the addition of inulin helps to eliminate the disease-causing bacteria, thus promoting healthy weight gain. Chicks switched to inulin gain weight rapidly, much to the ranchers' delight and, as an important consumer benefit, they are far less likely to be contaminated with disease-causing pathogens. The effect of such feeding on salmonella colonization was investigated by researchers at the Department of Veterinary Medicine, College of Agriculture, Osaka Prefecture University, Sakai, Japan.[21] Average numbers of *Salmonella enteritidis* in the chicks of the prebiotic group were significantly decreased compared with the control group. "Low-dose feeding of FOS in the diet of chicks . . . may result in reduced susceptibility to Salmonella colonization . . . ."

As I have discovered with my own patients, the end result is that with restoration of healthy populations of beneficial bacteria in the gastrointestinal tract, antibiotic-related side effects such as diarrhea and constipation as well as yeast infection can be minimized or even eliminated.

Inulin & Antibiotics

ANTIBIOTIC-RELATED CHILDHOOD DIARRHEA

Prebiotics as well as live bacterial cultures are both especially important to use with antibiotics for treatment of infantile acute diarrhea (by rotavirus or other agents), colitis, hospital-acquired and antibiotic-associated diarrheas.[22]

Indeed, most recently, pediatric researchers from Johns Hopkins University in Baltimore found that enhancing infants' populations of beneficial bacteria was shown to decrease incidences of diarrhea and diaper rash.[23] In the study, presented at a children's nutrition conference in 1998, the researchers gave 140 children, ages four to eighteen months, baby formula supplemented with high doses of beneficial bacterial, lactobacilli and bifidobacteria, found in the small intestine and colon, respectively. The result was a 20 percent reduction in diaper rash, fewer loose stools and less constipation among the supplemented babies.

In another study from *Clinical Pediatrics*, the effects of yogurt (containing beneficial bacteria) and Neomycin-kaopectate as treatment of infantile diarrhea were compared among 45 infants aged one to twenty-seven months who did not receive the additional yogurt. Infants treated with yogurt recovered more rapidly.[24]

ANTIBIOTIC-RELATED CONSTIPATION

Constipation is an ailment encountered often in elderly people, as well as in persons of all ages, especially when it is antibiotic-related.

Inulin & Antibiotics

Let me give you case examples from my own practice.

Michael, Geraldine and Linda all have one thing in common: multiple back surgeries and chronic pain that was so intense they required daily, potent opioid therapy. The result was decreased pain and concomitant constipation due to the opioid drugs which frequently disturbed bowel function. In fact, with opioid therapy, constipation is even expected as characterized by hardening of the stool with less frequent defecation.

Each had tried various laxative preparations, using them singly at high doses and in combination. They even tried powdered vitamin C, which is a generally effective laxative when taken by the teaspoon (two to five grams) every thirty minutes. The vitamin C worked somewhat effectively but was fairly harsh, too. High dosages of magnesium chloride helped but could not normalize their bowel function.

Each patient was then asked to take inulin—two grams three times a day—for two weeks. The results were very encouraging with less gas and straining, and a more normal appearance of their stools with greater frequency.

My findings are backed by scientific research. A study was initiated to test the effects of lactose or inulin on the bowel habits of constipated elderly patients and to correlate these effects with several variables measured in feces such as microflora.[25] Groups of 15 and 10 patients received lactose and inulin, respectively, for a period of 19 days. The dose was 20 grams per day (g/d) from days 1 to 8, was gradually increased to 40 g/d from days 9 to 11 and was kept at this dose from days 12 to 19. There was considerable interindividual variation with this kind of dietary intervention. However, overall, inulin significantly increased bifidobacteria populations and decreased populations of disease-causing bacteria such as enterococci and enterobacteria. In individuals consuming lactose, however, there was a noticeable increase in the population of enterococci and a decrease in lactobacilli. The researchers said that inulin showed a better laxative effect than lactose and reduced functional constipation with only mild discomfort.

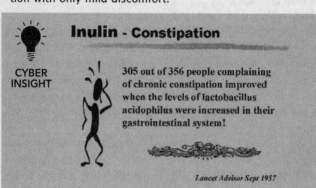

CYBER INSIGHT

Inulin - Constipation

305 out of 356 people complaining of chronic constipation improved when the levels of lactobacillus acidophilus were increased in their gastrointestinal system!

Lancet Advisor Sept 1957

In another study, 305 of 356 cases of chronic constipation responded to improvement in *Lactobacillus acidophilus* population.[26]

Finally, successfully bolstering lactobacillus populations was followed by relief of constipation resulting from a variety of triggering conditions such as mucous colitis, irritable colon, and idiopathic ulcerative colitis.[27] Additional studies dating to the 1920s and 1930s also bolster the use of prebiotics for boosting populations of friendly bacteria and reducing constipation.[28, 29]

In short, diarrhea, constipation, and loss of beneficial bacterial populations as a side-effect of antibiotic regimens can all be overcome with use of inulin.[30, 31]

HOW TO USE INULIN WITH ANTIBIOTICS

It is critical that consumers begin their use of inulin during antibiotic therapy and continue such for at least two weeks post-therapy. Take one to four 1,000 mg tablets of inulin three times a day with meals and *Inulin & Antibiotics* glass of water. Inulin is also available in five-gram packets. Many of my patients prefer the powdered form which they mix with their favorite juice in the morning, afternoon and/or evening. Adjust your dosage, accordingly, up or down, for optimal results to enhance your bowel movements.

For infants and children under twelve, reduce the dosage by half.

For very young children under age five, reduce the dosage to a quarter or less of the adult dosage, and adjust upward as required. Inulin tablets may be broken up and added to their favorite juice. Or simply use a quarter-pack of powdered inulin.

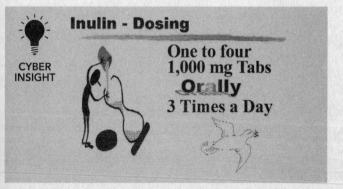

CYBER INSIGHT

Inulin - Dosing

One to four
1,000 mg Tabs
Orally
3 Times a Day

Inulin has a sweet pleasant taste and is highly palatable. It may also be added to applesauce, pudding or your favorite cherry soup recipe (kids love cherry—the preferred flavor of any cough syrup or liquid antibiotic).

FIVE

Enhance Immune Function & Resistance to Infectious Disease

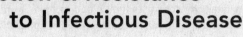

CAN YOU READ EGYPTIAN HIEROGLYPHICS? If so, you would learn some fascinating secrets of ancient Egyptian medicine. In *Science and Secrets of Early Medicine*—which makes for fascinating reading for all persons interested in ancient medical practices—we learn that many ancient Egyptian prescriptions included droppings from the common fly and pelicans, excrement from lizards and the Nile crocodile, even dung of the gazelle, as well as human urine.[32]

Even now, we find North African nomads often treat dysentery with bits of fresh horse or camel dung.

What do we make of this dung therapy? Were the ancient Egyptians and their modern descendents out of their minds?

Not at all!

As explained in *Science and Secrets of Early Medicine*, we now know "that bacteria living in the human body release their excretory products into the faeces and urine, which therefore are rich in antibiotic substances."*

Well, today, we have a more palatable alternative: inulin.

Very recently, researchers from the University of Paris dramatically demonstrated the positive impact that a healthy population of friendly flora in the body have on immunity in a

---

* *Even today in western medicine, as grotesque as it may sound, medical doctors sometimes use maggots as part of standard protocol to clear up wound infections and rid them of bad bacteria.*

report in the *American Journal of Clinical Nutrition*.[33] What's more, they found that the effect was sustained.

In this study, 28 healthy volunteers were given milk to drink with or without the two major friendly bacteria in the gut, *Lactobacillus acidophilus* and *Bifidobacterium bifidum*. Three weeks later, the scientists took blood samples from the volunteers and intentionally contaminated them with disease-causing *E. Coli*, a bacteria commonly found in beef that causes severe vomiting, nausea, kidney failure and some deaths, particularly in children and the elderly. The percentage of white blood cells known as phagocytes (which ingest bacteria and cell debris) that attacked and gobbled up *E. Coli* was 40 to 80 percent higher in the persons receiving the friendly strains of bacteria but not in those drinking plain milk. Six weeks after the volunteers ceased drinking their milk with friendly bacteria, their phagocyte activity remained far higher than when they began the study.

Friendly bacteria help the body to subdue many bacterial enemies—including *Candida albicans*, *Escherichia coli*, *Salmonella typhosa*, *Staphylococcus aureus*, shigella, clostridium, *Bacillus cereus*, *Streptococcus faecalis*, and *Campylobacter jejuni*. They do so via their natural secretions which act as natural antibiotics (especially when our levels of the B vitamins folic acid and riboflavin are adequate) and by population displacement of unfriendly strains.

Thus, they really rev up our immune function.

As a doctor, I know how important inulin can be to my patients' immune function. Bifidobacteria are the most predominating intestinal flora in infants. Children with high numbers of bifidobacteria resist enteric infections very effectively. In fact, the feeding of bifidobacteria-containing dairy products has been used to treat infections in Japanese children with success.

This is critical information for adults and children alike, by the way. For example, we know that breast-fed babies get fewer infections. When a baby is born, the intestines are virtually sterile and free of microorganisms. Then, within days ensues a landgrab, the likes of which haven't been seen since the days of the Wild West. Friendly and unfriendly germs alike rush in to take over the empty land of the child's intestine. By the fourth to seventh day, breast-fed babies' intestines generally have enough friendly bifidobacteria from their mother's milk to keep the bad guys at bay. Unfortunately, infant formula cannot provide the same beneficial bacteria. Thus, infants given formula tend to be overrun by bad bacteria.

Enhance Immune Function & Resistance to Infectious Disease

This is similar to what happens with antibiotics, too. Only in this case, antibiotics wipe out populations of friendly bacterial inhabitants of portions of the intestines to set up the land grab. In this case, taking inulin can position the good guys on our side to form an impenetrable barrier to keep out the bad actors.

We also know that, generally, compared to healthy children and adults, the elderly have very low counts of bifidobacteria. Unfortunately, as bifidobacteria numbers drop, there is a corresponding increase in the numbers of toxic species of *Clostridium perfringens* detected in the elderly. This can cause all sorts of problems, as *C. perfringens* produces a host of undesirable substances including toxins and volatile amines that can be potentially cancer causing. Yet, adults who bolster their population of friendly bacteria have demonstrated substantial decreases in clostridium counts as well as an increase in bifidobacterium counts. This translates into better health as we age.

Boosting the body's populations of friendly bacteria boosts its anti-infectious properties. Medical journalist Dr. Morton Walker reports in his book *Secrets of Long Life* that *Lacotbacilli Acidophilus* contains several other powerful anti-microbial compounds such as acidolin, acidophyllin, acidolphin, lactocidin, and bacteriocin. These germ-fighting bacterial compounds have been proven to eradicate campylobacter, listeria, staphylococci, chronic yeast infections, herpes and flu viruses. For example, in a test tube experimental study, acidophyllin, one of the antibacterial components of acidophilus, caused a 50 percent inhibition in growth of 27 different types of bacterial species including 23 common pathogens.[34, 35, 36, 37]

CYBER INSIGHT

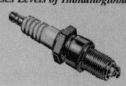

Lactobacillus Rhamnosus

- *Activates Natural Killer Cells*
- *Improves Macrophage Phagocyte Function*
- *Increases Levels of Immunoglobulins*

SPECIAL REPORT: INULIN AND *LACTOBACILLI RHAMNOSUS*

There are many different kinds of lactobacilli species. One of the most important, exciting strains is *Lactobacilli Rhamnosus*. Leading Canadian bacteriologist Dr. Edward Brochu, of the Institute Rosell of Montreal, reports that this particular strain has been shown to have very exciting immune-boosting properties including the following:

✦ Activation of natural killer cells to reduce cancer risk.

✦ Improved resistance to listeria monocytogenes which can cause encephalitis.

✦ Improved phagocytic activity by the body's white blood cells called macrophages.

✦ Increased levels of infection-fighting immunoglobulins.

"*Lactobacillus rhamnosus* may be considered as one of the most important lactobacilli, if not the best," says Dr. Brochu.

Inulin, of course, helps to boost the body's levels of all resident beneficial strains—including *Lactobacillus rhamnosus*.

BOOSTING POPULATIONS OF FRIENDLY BACTERIA PROTECTS AGAINST ADDITIONAL MALADIES

Vaginitis

Vaginitis is often caused by a tiny, one-celled organism called trichomonas. Another cause may be elevated populations of pathogenic organisms called gardnerella. Symptoms include itching and irritation of the vagina and swelling and redness of the vulva.

Boosting friendly bacterial populations offers protection against vaginitis. Not only is its occurrence and recurrence reduced, women can avoid having to repeatedly rely on potentially dangerous medical drugs commonly used to treat this condition. In contrast to conventional therapy without adjuvant prebiotics, simultaneous treatment with inulin can help to protect against reinfection.[38]

Enhance Immune Function & Resistance to Infectious Disease

We know that a decrease in women's lactobacillus populations is associated with increased risk for vaginitis. In a study of 12 women with non-specific chronic vaginitis, it was found that women were most likely to be symptom-free when their populations of lactobacilli were highest. As the lactobacilli populations decreased, bacterial pathogens were commonly isolated, indicating a disturbed vaginal ecology.[39]

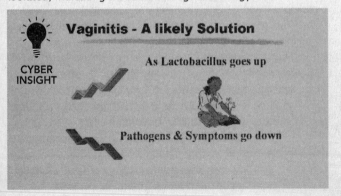

CYBER INSIGHT

Vaginitis - A likely Solution

As Lactobacillus goes up

Pathogens & Symptoms go down

In another study, samples of vaginal fluid from 60 women indicated that as the population of lactobacillus went down, the population of bacterial pathogens went up.[40] These findings were reconfirmed in another observational study when vaginal fluid from 53 women with nonspecific vaginitis and without the condition was analyzed and the populations of pathogenic bacteria were found to be elevated in women with the condition.[41]

Supplementation with inulin to boost the body's overall populations of lactobacillus can help to reduce chronic vaginitis.

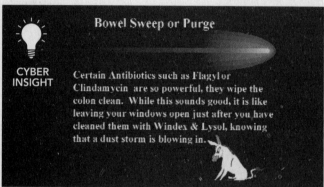

Bowel Sweep or Purge

CYBER INSIGHT

Certain Antibiotics such as Flagyl or Clindamycin are so powerful, they wipe the colon clean. While this sounds good, it is like leaving your windows open just after you have cleaned them with Windex & Lysol, knowing that a dust storm is blowing in.

Indeed, such supplementation with inulin may be preferable to a course of metronidazole (Flagyl), which may kill both trichomonas and gardnerella. Metronidazole is known by doctors and pharmacists alike as the ultimate "bowel sweeper," taking everything—including friendly bacteria—with it.

Flagyl, made by G.D. Searle, is one of the most widely prescribed antibiotics. It was the first effective drug against vaginal infections (trichomonas), for which it is still widely used. By the mid-1970s, it was prescribed more than two million times annually.[42]

"Noteworthy" incidence of breast cancer in rats has been found following dosing with metronidazole. The drug is characterized as having "considerable carcinogenic potential."[43]

A subsequent animal study also reported "significant" excesses of breast cancer.[44] While two short-term and inadequate human studies found no excesses of breast cancer, the animal evidence raises a clear warning.[45, 46]

On the other hand with inulin we have a safe alternative or complement to antibiotic use.

In one study of 94 patients with non-specific vaginitis, treatment with a supplement to increase the body's populations of beneficial lactobacillus resulted in a decrease of pathogens and increase in the population of normal lactobacilli.[47] Vaginal purity and vaginal pH also returned to normal. A cure or at least marked improvement in symptoms was documented in 80 percent of patients. Boosting the body's own healing response by restoring its population of friendly bacteria protects against reinfection and has a decided advantage over antibiotic therapy alone.

Enhance Immune Function & Resistance to Infectious Disease

Vaginitis: The Data

CYBER INSIGHT

444 women with trichomoniasis vaginalis
Treatment: Prebiotic therapy (No antibioitics)

Results: 96.2% (427 women) cured
Follow-up @ 1 year

In a second study, 444 women with *trichomoniasis vaginalis* were treated with a supplement to raise populations of friendly bacteria.[48] One year later, 427 (96.2%) were followed up, and 92.5% of them were found to be cured of clinical symptoms, while the remaining 7.5% had either a positive slide or culture.

In another clinical report, 20 patients reported that they

cured their candida vulvovaginitis with preparations designed to enhance their populations of friendly bacteria.[49]

Cystitis and Lower Urinary Tract Infections (UTIs)

Despite ever–improving antibiotic therapy, 10 percent of the population is affected by infections of the urinary tract, most often afflicting the bladder as well. Acute primary or secondary cystitis usually involves an infectious inflammation of the bladder mucosa. As in all urinary tract infections, the characteristic quartet of bacterial pathogens which appear again and again is also encountered here: E. coli, Enterococci, Proteus bacteria and Staphylococcus aureus, in a mono or polyinfection.

Cystitis can develop in the kidneys or via the urethra and appendages, spreading systemically. Due to their short urethra, women are more liable to be afflicted with types of ascending infections. Contributory factors are colds, urinary retention and changes in the local environment due to hormonal factors as well as prior damage by allergic cystitis, radiation cystitis or toxic cystitis (effects of chemical substances).

In addition to measures as bed rest, fluid intake and analgesics, the causative agents respond to specific chemotherapy.

Cystitis and UTIs tend to become chronic, especially if the mucosa was damaged previously. Chronic cystitis and UTIs often proceed intermittently. The deeper layers of the bladder wall are usually also involved in the inflammatory process.

Prebiotics such as inulin are also important to use with antibiotics when being treated for urinary tract infections (UTIs)—as the same medicines that eradicate infectious agents cause imbalances in the bacterial populations that protect against UTIs. This leads to risk of re-infection. Prebiotics help to repopulate the body's beneficial bacteria that protect against UTIs.

By supporting the body's population of L. acidophilus, prebiotics help to restore a normal population of gram-negative bacteria following administration of broad-spectrum antibiotics.[50]

Candida

If you're feeling "sick all over" and if you've been regularly using antibiotics, you could be suffering from complications of yeast syndrome. A lot of my women patients suffer from candidiasis, also known as yeast syndrome, when they first come to see me. Fortunately, with use of holistic healing pathways, including use of inulin, I can usually help them eliminate candida from their lives altogether.

An overgrowth in the gastrointestinal tract of the usually benign yeast (or fungus), *Candida albicans* is now becoming recognized as a complex medical syndrome called *chronic candidiasis* or the *yeast syndrome*. Many women have yeast syndrome but don't even know it is the reason they feel "sick all over." Yet, even women who know they suffer from yeast syndrome often live with this debilitating condition for years, because their doctors are unable to provide them with a safe and effective healing program.

Enhance Immune Function & Resistance to Infectious Disease

The typical patient with the yeast syndrome is young and female. Indeed, women are eight times more likely to experience the yeast syndrome than men. They have usually been on estrogen drugs such as birth-control pills and have been given a higher than normal number of prescriptions for antibiotics, most notably tetracycline and metronidazole and topical creams such as erythromycin.

Prolonged antibiotic use is believed to be the most important factor in the development of chronic candidiasis. Antibiotics suppress the immune system and the normal intestinal bacteria that prevent yeast overgrowth, strongly promoting the proliferation of candida.

Normally, friendly bacterial help to keep the candida organism in check. But when their populations are decreased, the candida germs gain control.

That means the gastrointestinal tract of candida sufferers often must be recultivated with healthy bacteria. Products that stimulate *L. acidophilus* or *B. bifidum* can help immensely as part of a comprehensive program that addresses the whole person. Inulin is a natural supplement to aid in restoring such populations that can then enhance the healing response so that my patients may get past the chronic infectious state.

Childhood Allergies

Although we don't have a lot of evidence on beneficial bacteria and children's allergies, in one study on childhood food allergies, it was found that a deficiency of *Lactobacillus Acidophilus* and *Bifidobacteria* combined with overgrowth of *Enterobacteriaceae* was common to *all* cases of allergy among a group of children.[51] Thus, again, inulin could prove very helpful. This is backed by my own clinical experience wherein children with food allergies tend to improve markedly once we get them on a daily dose of inulin (usually as part of their cereal or juice).

SIX

Inulin & Dyspepsia

FED UP WITH CHRONIC GAS, NAUSEA, belching, bloating and even vomiting? Ask your doctor for help and he or she will probably respond by first taking your history and performing a physical examination. Your doctor will view the esophagus and check for any types of perforations as well as test you for the presence of ulcer-causing *Helicobacter pylori*. If the finding for *H. pylori* is positive, the patient usually will be treated with antibiotics as well as drugs to suppress symptoms rather than initiate the healing response.

These drugs include various antibiotics, Pepto-Bismol, and the new class of proton pump inhibitors such as omeprazole

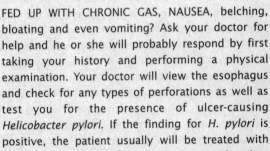

Symptom Suppression vs Healing

CYBER INSIGHT

In Dyspepsia, it is common to give expensive drugs that suppress symptoms such as Proton Pump Inhibitors (Prilosec, Prevacid, Aciphex, or H2-Blockers (Tagamet, Zantac, Pepcid, Axid) or anticholinergics, smooth muscle drugs such as Bentyl, Levsin, Donnatal. This is treatment without insight and unlikely to enhance the healing response.

(Prilosec®) or H-2 blockers like cimetadine (Tagamet®), raniti-dine (Zantac®), and famotidine (Pepcid®).

All of these may be somewhat helpful but very often the indigestion persists, meaning that we really haven't solved the underlying causative agent.

If the findings for *H. pylori* are negative, the doctor usually writes out a prescription for a drug that will relieve symptoms temporarily or give a drug that interferes with the natural GI acid secretions, or tell the patient to simply take more Tums or another OTC antacid. If the doctor is still not sure what's causing a patient's indigestion, the patient may be subjected to an upper gastrointestinal tract x-ray or the doctor may use an endoscope to rule out stomach cancer or look more specifically for non-bacterially caused ulcers.

Most typically, doctors recommend the H-2 receptor antagonists. These drugs which are available over the counter work by occupying sites on the surface of gastric cells. These sites are called histamine H-2 receptors. When specific types of histamines (a type of substance composed from ammonia) attach to them, these receptors signal the stomach cells to secrete various chemicals such as hydrochloric acid that help to digest food. By taking up residence on these receptors the drug prevents histamines from occupying the spaces on these receptors and turning on these cells. The volume of acidic secretions in the stomach is reduced. This temporarily reduces your symptoms. But this is only a temporary solution, since excess acid secretions are not the cause of indigestion but merely a symptom.

We have other drugs we can use. Drugs such as antacids (Mylanta, Maalox, or Tums) can help to neutralize stomach acidity by adding a buffering mineral such as calcium. Meanwhile, motility enhancement drugs are also used. These include cisapride (Propulsid®) or metoclo-pramide (Reglan®). These work by stimulating gastric emptying of both solids and liquids.

Although most often, their side effects or complications are mild, they may be quite serious in some patients. For example, people using famotidine or ranitidine may be more likely to suffer from mild to severe headaches, dizziness, constipation and diarrhea. (Especially in the case of the last two complications—constipation and diarrhea—that's why inulin is so important to add to patients' drug regimens.)

The complications from cimetidine may be more serious. While not cancer-causing in rodents, cimetidine does alter the body's metabolism of estrogen, causing gynecomastia in men.[52] These estrogenic effects are consistent with a single report of breast cancer *Inulin & Dyspepsia* in a man who had been treated with cimetadine.[53] "After being on [on the drug] for eight months . . . he was found to have a hard malignant mass replacing his right breast." Clearly, human studies on this drug are overdue, especially as it is in very common use.

The Physicians' Desk Reference warns that serious heart arrhythmias have been reported in patients who are using cisapride with other medications, including some common antibiotics. The drug could potentially impair fertility, according to experimental studies.

Metoclopramide can cause mental depression including suicidal tendencies, Parkinsonian-like symptoms, and tardive dyskinesia; other complications include restlessness, drowsiness, fatigue and lassitude; levels of a hormone called prolactin may be increased which may increase women's risk for breast cancer.

As for omeprazole (Prilosec), it may be cancer-causing, based on experimental studies reported on in *The Physicians' Desk Reference*. In two 24-month studies, omeprazole at daily doses approximately four to three-hundred-fifty-two times the human dose produced gastric cell cancers in a dose-related manner in both male and female rats; the incidence of this effect was markedly higher in female rats, which had higher blood levels of omeprazole. Gastric cancers seldom occur in the untreated rat. In addition, abnormal cell growth was present in all treated groups of both sexes. An unusual primary malignant tumor in the stomach was seen in one rat. No similar tumor was seen in male or female rats treated for two years. For this strain of rat no similar tumor has been noted historically, but a finding involving only one tumor is difficult to interpret. A 78-week mouse carcinogenicity study of omeprazole did not show increased tumor occurrence, but the study was not conclusive.

For a complete break-out of the safety of these commonly prescribed drugs, see Table 6.1 (next page).

What's more, very often, these quick fixes offer no permanent solution. The problem is that the next time you eat you will once again end up suffering from uncomfortable, sometimes embarrassing symptoms of indigestion.

Using typical prescription or over the counter drugs offers a temporary fix but doesn't attack your problem at the source. Your doctor has treated your symptoms but without initiating the healing process. The real solution to indigestion or irritable bowel syndrome is to understand the cause and address the problem at its root.

When more serious illnesses are ruled out, doctors practicing complementary medicine prefer to treat their patients with natural therapies such as dietary changes and nutritional supplements. That is why inulin is being recognized and applauded as a welcome addition to health enhancement. Inulin is still new to most doctors in the United States. Along with the Hippocratic Oath, "Do no harm," inulin is safe and well worth giving people who suffer from dyspepsia. It's a unique way of helping people with indigestion or irritable bowel syndrome that works. Inulin is a natural cure that will, in fact, correct your indigestion problem or irritable bowel syndrome at its source.

Mild, occasional indigestion is generally transient and self-limiting without the need of medical care. But when indigestion becomes a chronic problem that accompanies practically every meal, then you have a serious problem. Often overlooked by

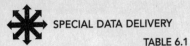 SPECIAL DATA DELIVERY

TABLE 6.1
Safe Shopper's Chart:
Inulin vs. Medical Drugs for Indigestion

Typically Prescribed Drug	Adverse Reactions/Possible Chronic Toxicity
Inulin (InuFlora)	None.
Magnesium hydroxide (Maalox, Milk of Magnesia, Mylanta, Tums)	No significant adverse or chronic effects Possible drug interactions.
Cimetidine (Tagamet®)	Headaches, headaches, gynecomastia, impotence, decreased white blood cell counts, congested liver, increases in plasma creatinine, experimental evidence of possible carcinogenic effect.
Cisapride (Propulsid®)	Headache, diarrhea, abdominal pain, fatal irregular heartbeat, dyspepsia, urinary tract infection, increased frequency of urination, abnormal vision. Use this drug only after a complete EKG.
Famotidine (Pepcid®)	Headache, dizziness, constipation, diarrhea. Possibly arrhythmia, palpitations, tinnitus.
Metoclopramide (Reglan®)	Restlessness, drowsiness, fatigue and lassitude, depression, dystonia tardive dyskinesia, elevated prolactin (possibly increased cancer risk), gynecomastia, impotence.
Omeprazole (Prilosec®)	Abdominal pain, diarrhea, headache, possible carcinogenicity based on experimental studies.
Ranitidine (Zantac®)	Severe headache, dizziness, insomnia, vertigo, arrhythmia, constipation, diarrhea, nausea, increases in liver SGPT values, blood count changes

What is Indigestion?

Upwards of 100 million Americans live with and suffer from chronic gastrointestinal problems. They may be of any age or background, since gastrointestinal problems cut across all barriers of age and economic class. In fact, next to the common cold, gastrointestinal problems account for more absences from work and more visits to the doctor than any other condition. Symptoms may be continuous, with daily pain and discomfort, or they may subside for days or weeks at a time only to come back without any seeming provocation whatsoever.

If you feel gaseous or bloated, suffer excessive flatulence, constipation, nausea or vomit after meals on a regular basis, then you may be suffering from chronic indigestion or other eating disorders such as irritable bowel syndrome, bulimia or anorexia.

Known medically as dyspepsia, indigestion is characterized by upper abdominal discomfort and pain with bloating and fullness after eating. Other symptoms may include belching, bloating, burping, heartburn, loss of appetite, regurgitation, early feeling of fullness, perhaps even nausea and vomiting. The symptoms typically occur one to two hours after a meal and may be temporarily improved by taking antacids. About one-third of Americans today suffer from chronic indigestion.*

In fact, such symptoms may also underlie some of the early signs of eating disorders such as anorexia and bulimia, which are being diagnosed now at alarming rates. Be sure to consult a qualified health professional if you suspect anorexia or bulimia.

the medical profession is that a significant cause of indigestion and even irritable bowel syndrome is *not* necessarily oversecretion of hydrochloric acid but the result of inability to digest and assimilate food—particularly when we have experienced constipation, diarrhea, and mineral depletion on a long-term basis.

Indigestion is often the result of our old friend, dysbiosis. Lactobacilli are indispensable to healthy digestion because of their ability to produce digestive enzymes including proteases, beta-galactosidase, and lipases that digest protein, sugar and fats, respectively.[54, 55] This in turn produces acids that support a healthy pH and enhance nutrient assimilation.

Inulin & Dyspepsia

Another key benefit is that healthy bacterial populations stimulate peristalsis, the wave-like motion of the smooth muscles of the digestive system as they expand and contract and move along food as it is being digested. Very often, poor peristalsis is the result of inadequate fiber and fluids. Inulin aids peristalsis both as a bulking agent and by liquefying the contents of the colon.

The large intestine is an anaerobic environment and home to the digestive system's highest concentration of bacteria with 100 billion to 1,000 billion microorganisms per tablespoon. When food has reached the large intestine, it is very loose and watery. Its nutrients have been absorbed, and the body must now transport out the waste. To do so, this liquid watery mass must be reconverted into a solid and then excreted. It is key that this process occur quickly, for otherwise the wastes putrefy and produce toxic, often carcinogenic substances that can cause chronic disease including cancer. The large intestine's population of beneficial bacteria help to accelerate this process as well as offer protection against toxicity. They stimulate peristalsis and prevent conversion of toxins into carcinogens. Their healthy population prevents pathogenic strains from taking up residence.

And if you are lactose intolerance, here's another bonus. Inulin's beneficial effects on friendly bacterial populations may help alleviate lactose intolerance caused by deficiency of the enzyme lactase. That is because friendly bacterial strains like *Lactobacillus acidophilus* produce enormous quantities of lactase that can help to digest the milk sugar lactose more fully. This in turn should help to relieve the bad breath, bloating, gas formation and stomach cramps associated with lactose intolerance.[56, 57]

IRRITABLE BOWEL SYNDROME

Increasing the body's overall lactobacillus levels may be useful in treating irritable bowel syndrome, according to a report in *The Lancet*.[58] What's more, inulin is a fiber, another aspect with benefits for persons suffering from irritable bowel syndrome. When using inulin as a fiber, be sure to take about eight to fifteen grams daily. The evidence that fiber is strongly therapeutic for irritable bowel syndrome span decades and is fairly strong.[59, 60] But the dual properties of inulin as a fiber *and* prebiotic could make it the superior alternative.

Let me give you an example or two from my own practice. Dee was 49 and diagnosed with fibromyalgia with a concomitant diagnosis of irritable bowel syndrome, from which she had suffered for years. Within one week of beginning to use inulin, she felt less spasms, bloating, and gas. She can talk again without gurgling. Food is tasting better because there seems to be less acid in her stomach.

Dee jokes that she has received the Jerusalem blessing. She is now more open to changing other aspects of her diet and lifestyle that she didn't want to address previously—for example, consuming fewer diet soft drinks and coffee and stopping the smoking habit. There has been a change in Dee. Her healing response has been sparked.

Brenda suffered from fibromyalgia, a condition with chronic muscle pain. Like many fibromyalgia sufferers, Brenda also was suffering irritable bowel syndrome. The symptoms were always bothersome and beginning to wear her down. Her bowel patterns were so irregular and unpredictable that she was afraid to even go out. She avoided milk and dairy products, fearing they would worsen her condition. She also avoided high fat foods and sugar and was afraid of spices. But her greatest fear was having to take antibiotics. She could not tolerate them.

Fortunately, when I began Brenda on inulin, her tolerance was excellent. It took a little while for the inulin to take effect, but within about two weeks she began feeling differ-ent. What she noticed was a gradual change in her self confidence. She began going out to eat again.

Inulin & Dyspepsia

Interestingly, inulin improved Brenda's mood, too. She began to wake with more energy. I believe that a pathway was opened that enhanced Brenda's body's own healing response. Perhaps too, by improving her digestion, her levels of serotonin, a feel-good hormone that is intimately associated with digestive processes, increased. This is a promising area of research with inulin that I certainly want to see more research done on.

NUTRIENT ASSIMILATION
AND MINERAL UTILIZATION

Very much part of healthy digestion is nutrient assimilation and, specifically, mineral utilization. Inulin presents fantastic benefits in this area. The acidification of fermented dairy prod-ucts by bifidobacteria and their slight proteolytic activity may help to increase the amount of calcium absorbed by the body as well as improve digestibility. Inulin and oligofructose signif-icantly increase the intestinal absorption of calcium, iron and magnesium, as demonstrated and confirmed by several exper-imental studies. By enhancing mineral utilization it may even help women patients to ward off osteoporosis.

In an experimental study from the Nutritional Science Center, Bioscience Laboratories, Saitama, Japan, researchers have shown that inulin, which is a FOS, increases the absorption of calcium from the large intestine of healthy rats.[61] "The net calcium absorption in . . . the fructooligosaccharides diet was greater than that in [the] . . . control diet. . . . Dietary fructooligosaccharides enhanced calcium absorption and prevented . . . changes . . . such as decreases in bone calcium content and bone mineral density . . . ."

Other researchers from the Departments of Pharmacology, School of Dentistry, Showa University, Shinagawa-ku, Tokyo, Japan, have also observed such beneficial effects on the body's retention of key minerals.[62] "These results suggest that the increased true calcium absorption and balance produced by FOS feeding might improve bone calcification."

Subsequent experiments have further revealed that the increased calcium absorption results in increased bone-mineral density.

This means that the increased absorption effectively results in building up the body's calcium reserves. This may be particularly beneficial for menopausal women, as recently demonstrated in an unpublished experimental study model in which calcium uptake from food was improved and bone-mineral density increased when FOS was given to female rodents no longer producing youthful levels of estrogen.

Children, especially young women, can benefit from inulin. We also know from unpublished industry data that the intake of 15 grams per day of inulin significantly increases the absorption of calcium in teenagers. In yet another industry study where healthy adult volunteers were given 40 grams a day of inulin, a significant increase in calcium absorption was observed as well. Magnesium absorption also seemed to be enhanced.

This is an important finding, as it is in this particular period of life that humans build up their calcium reserve. The higher the peak bone mass becomes at this period of life, the more the probability for occurrence of osteoporosis in the future is reduced.

These results, when taken all together, provide promising evidence that inulin increases mineral absorption in humans and could therefore actively contribute to the prevention of osteoporosis.

But there's more benefit when it comes to enhanced nutrient utilization. In the human large intestine, bifidobacteria synthesize vitamins that are slowly absorbed in the body. Bifidobacteria are known to produce thiamin, riboflavin, and vitamins B_6, B_{12}, and K.[63, 64] Bifidobacteria can also synthesize amino acids for absorption in the gut. Adaptation of the gastrointestinal tract with bifidus enhances nitrogen retention while resulting in a 400 percent increase of vitamin B_6 content in stools.

Inulin & Dyspepsia

This is really important. We now know that many of the problems associated with aging such as senility, depression, loss of energy and even atheroslcerosis are sometimes caused by low levels of the B vitamins. And without proper bacteria to help produce these important nutrients, our bodies simply can't manufacture enough of these vitamins. That's why using inulin to reinvigorate populations of friendly vitamin B complex-producing bacteria is so beneficial to all persons but especially the elderly.

Even aching joints and bones may be helped. That is because lactobacilli help the body to produce vitamin K. This vitamin helps to build strong bones. A lack of vitamin K may predispose the body to osteoporosis-related joint damage.

SEVEN

Help for High Cholesterol & Blood Lipids

HEALTH-CONSCIOUS PEOPLE RECOGNIZE that high levels of both cholesterol and triglycerides increase their risk for heart disease. Unfortunately, millions of Americans suffer from high blood levels of each. While medical drugs may help to reduce cholesterol and triglyceride levels, their side effects may make them less desirable than a safe natural medicine such as inulin.

What is cholesterol? Cholesterol is not a fat but it is closely related to fat. It is a chemical that is an essential component in the structure of cells and is also involved in the formation of important hormones. If your diet contained no cholesterol your liver would still produce all the cholesterol you need.

However, high levels of a particular kind of cholesterol called low density lipoprotein (LDL or "bad" cholesterol) can contribute to coronary artery disease in which the blood vessels are narrowed by deposits of a fatty tissue called atheromas, which are comprised largely of cholesterol. Narrowing of the heart's coronary arteries by patches of atheroma can cause angina. This also increases the risk of an artery becoming blocked by a blood clot, leading to a heart attack or stroke.

On the other hand, your body also produces high density lipoproteins (HDLs, "good" cholesterol) which are quickly transported from the bloodstream and do not form atheroma deposits in the arteries.

TRIGLYCERIDES: ANOTHER
HEART DISEASE RISK FACTOR

What many people don't realize, however, is that triglycerides, a type of fat, are also now thought to be associated with increased risk for heart disease.

Previously major changeable risk factors for heart attack included smoking, high blood cholesterol, high blood pressure and physical inactivity. According to a study published in *Circulation*, however, high blood levels of the fat triglyceride may need to be added to the list.[65] Elevated triglycerides may be a consequence of other diseases, such as diabetes. Like cholesterol, triglyceride levels can be detected with a blood test.

Researchers say that in middle-aged and older white men, a high level of triglycerides—the chemical form in which most fat exists in food as well as in the body—may mean a higher risk for heart attack. Therefore, the scientists say, high blood levels of triglycerides should be considered an independent risk factor for heart attack. In the study, men with the highest levels of triglycerides were more than twice as likely to have a heart attack when compared to those with the lowest triglyceride levels.

"So far our study appears to provide the strongest evidence that higher triglyceride levels are related to increased risk of ischemic heart disease in men independent of other major risk factors such as total cholesterol and HDL (high-density lipoprotein) cholesterol," says lead investigator of the study Jørgen Jeppesen, M.D., of the Epidemiological Research Unit, Copenhagen University Hospital, Denmark.

In an accompanying editorial, former American Heart Association President Antonio Gotto, M.D. says that while additional research is necessary to determine whether lowering triglyceride levels can reduce heart attack deaths, the findings make a compelling argument for measuring triglyceride levels as part of an evaluation to determine an individual's risk for heart disease.

"The growing attention to high levels of triglycerides and increased coronary heart disease risk is encouraging to veterans of the 'triglyceride wars,'" says Gotto, dean of the Cornell University Medical School, New York City. "It's also in agreement with another trend in heart attack risk management, namely, the concept of global risk assessment."

Triglycerides are the form in which fat exists in meats, cheese, fish, nuts, vegetable oils, and the greasy layer on the surface of soup stocks or in a pan in which bacon has been fried. In a healthy person, triglycerides and other fatty substances are normally moved into the liver and into storage cells to provide energy for later use.

Help for High Cholesterol & Blood Lipids

High levels of triglycerides can influence the size, density distribution and composition of LDL (low-density lipoprotein) cholesterol—the "bad" cholesterol—leading to smaller, denser LDL particles, which are more likely to promote the obstructions in

CYBER INSIGHT

Quick Triglyceride Primer

Traditionally, people with less than 200 milligrams of triglycerides per deciliter (mg/dl) of blood are considered to have normal triglyceride levels. Between 200 and 400 mg/dl is borderline high; between 400 and 1,000 mg/dl is a high triglyceride level; and greater than 1,000 mg/dl is considered very high triglycerides. However, the normal range may require revision.

"A very interesting finding in our study was that people with triglyceride levels as low as 142 mg/dl were clearly at a higher risk of heart disease," says Jeppesen of the study published in *Circulation*. "We believe this is of substantial clinical interest since a triglyceride level of below 200 mg/dl is usually considered 'safe.'"

the blood vessels that trigger heart attack. An excess amount of triglycerides in blood is called hypertriglyceridemia.

In the study of 2,906 white men who were initially free of any heart disease, researchers found that during an eight year follow-up period, 229 men had a heart attack. By examining that group of men, the scientists found that heart attack risk increased in those with the highest levels of fasting triglycerides (measurements taken after 12 hours of fasting prior to the test).

"When the triglyceride levels were measured by the amounts of HDL cholesterol in the blood, a clearer picture emerged," says Jeppesen. "Even those who had high HDL levels, which are thought to protect against heart attack, were still found to be at higher risk for heart disease because of their triglyceride levels."

The American Heart Association says that changes in life habits—cutting down on calories, reducing saturated fat and cholesterol in the diet, reduced alcohol intake and a regular exercise program—can help in the treatment of hypertriglyceridemia, the technical name for elevated triglycerides.

PRESCRIPTION DRUGS FOR HIGH CHOLESTEROL

The pharmaceutical industry has developed many powerful medical drugs to help people lower cholesterol levels. In severe and life-threatening situations, medical drugs obviously have important uses.

But there are also two areas of concern. First, while we know that these drugs do lower cholesterol, the jury is out whether they still extend the life span of people with high cholesterol levels. Most studies have shown that people taking cholesterol-lowering drugs are at slightly higher overall risk of death than people not taking any cholesterol-lowering drugs. That is probably because these drugs tend to bind or inhibit the production of other essential nutrients necessary for heart health, or they have an adverse effect on brain neurotransmitters. More recently, encouraging results have been seen from clinical trials, and we are gaining greater faith in these drugs' ability to extend human life span. But I really think we want to use these drugs only when diet, lifestyle and natural healing pathways have been exhausted.

Indeed, in the area of preventive medicine, natural cholesterol-lowering agents are a viable choice. In particular, inulin selectively modifies the colon's bacterial populations and liver's formation of lipids.[66] Both of these, in turn, help the body to beneficially lower serum blood lipids. What's more, inulin is completely nontoxic and without any drug or nutrient interactions whatsoever.

Help for
High Cholesterol &
Blood Lipids

C.M. Williams of the Hugh Sinclair Unit of Human Nutrition, Department of Food Science and Technology, University of Reading, Reading, UK, notes that "convincing lipid-lowering effects of the fructooligosaccharide inulin have been demonstrated in animals . . . ."[67]

Inulin seems to work best if persons are consuming a diet high in carbohydrates. That is because we know that inulin works by inhibiting the liver's synthesis of fatty acids which are synthesized from some types of carbohydrates, and that this is the major pathway for its triglyceride-lowering effects. Biochemical studies with isolated liver cells have demonstrated that by altering gene expression inulin reduces the activity of the liver's key enzymes which are related to formation of fatty acids or assembling triglycerides. This pathway is relatively inactive in humans unless one is consuming a high carbohydrate diet. But if you like pastries, baked goods, candy and soft drinks or other forms of starch and carbohydrates such as rice and potatoes—then inulin could be your best friend, as it can really help to lower blood lipids including cholesterol and triglycerides.

Two clinical studies that fed inulin either in a breakfast cereal (9 grams per day) or as a powdered addition to beverages and meals (10 grams per day) reported similar reductions in fasting triglycerides (by 27 percent and 19 percent, respectively). In one of these studies, total and LDL cholesterol concentrations were also modestly reduced (by five percent and seven percent, respectively).

Most recently in 1999, researchers from the Chicago Center for Clinical Research conducted a randomized, double-blind crossover trial with two six-week periods. They found that inulin resulted in "significant" decrease in cholesterol, especially LDLs.[68]

In an experimental study, inulin reduced the most dangerous cholesterol fractions including not only serum triglycerides but very low-density lipoprotein cholesterol.

The studies indicate that the triglyceride–lowering effect takes about eight weeks to establish.

Of course, consuming a whole lot of inulin can really help. In one study, the addition of 10 percent inulin to a fat-rich diet reduced the post-meal serum triglyceride contents, as well as the serum cholesterol content, by more than 50 percent compared with control groups.

Well, that's an extreme case. But the point we're trying to make is that inulin, even in the moderate dosages we're recommending, can be very helpful when it comes to lowering not only serum cholesterol but triglycerides.

Of course, because inulin is so well tolerated, you could consume a whole lot more and enjoy truly miraculous cholesterol—and triglyceride-lowering benefits.

CYBER
INFO
SITE

How to Use Inulin for Cholesterol- and Triglyceride-lowering Effects

One great way to use inulin for its cholesterol- and triglyceride-lowering effects is to mix one or two heaping tablespoons of powdered inulin with orange juice. Not only do you receive all the benefits of inulin but also the antioxidant properties of orange juice, plus a generous amount of potassium, an essential mineral for cardiovascular health.

EIGHT

Cancer Prevention

A RECENT REPORT in *Nutrition Action Health Letter* notes that, "If you're not a smoker, the cancer that's most likely to kill you—other than breast or prostate—is cancer of the colon or rectum. In 1999, an estimated 94,700 Americans will be diagnosed with colon cancer and 34,700 with rectal cancer. Within ten years, 55 percent of them will die."[69]

But we have reason to be optimistic. We can prevent or markedly reduce our risk for colon cancers through our dietary habits. It is in the area of prevention of one of our most deadly cancers, that of the colon, that inulin offers stellar benefits. We don't think of the friendly bacteria in our gastrointestinal tract as important components of cancer prevention. Yet, healthy populations of friendly bacteria play many important roles in our body's quest to defend itself against malignant disease.[70, 71]

Take for example, beta glucuronidase, an enzyme that disrupts our ability to detoxify environmental chemicals and hormones, such as estrogen, that the body naturally produces. High levels of beta glucuronidase in the body appear to put people at risk for both breast and colon cancer.

However, a healthy flourishing population of friendly bacteria helps to displace unfriendly strains responsible for producing this enzyme.[72] Your protection against two prevalent, often deadly cancers is thereby enhanced.

Very recent research from the American Health Foundation, Valhalla, New York, indicates that inulin and oligofructose have a significant chemopreventive potential and can prevent formation of precancerous lesions (i.e., polyps) in the colon, markedly delaying or even preventing the cancer process. Inulin seems to be more effective than other FOS products with shorter chains of complex sugars in preventing lesion formation in the distal part of the colon, site of the highest cancer incidence in humans. This may be due to slower fermentation of the long-chain molecules, and, hence, greater bacterial activity in the distal part of the colon. Other experiments indicate that long-chain inulin is also able to delay the propagation phase of colon carcinogenesis in rats.

It was furthermore experimentally demonstrated that inulin inhibits the development of transplanted cancer cells. In such experiments, it also can reduce the development of chemically induced breast cancer in rats (see next page).

We don't know precisely how inulin exerts its anti-cancer benefits but believe that by enhancing populations of bifidobacteria, this may result in direct removal of procarcinogens, indirect removal of procarcinogens, or activation of the body's immune system. In one experimental study, it was shown that a particular strain of acidophilus could prevent tumor formation in rats challenged by a chemical carcinogen.[73] The researchers involved in the study postulate that the inhibition of cancer "may involve (a) inhibiting the growth of putrefactive bacteria and in turn reducing the production of N-nitroso compounds; (b) direct reduction of secondary nitrites and bile salts . . . and (c) stimulation of intraperitoneal macrophages and their enzymes which may play a role in the antitumor effect . . ."

Tumor suppression via the body's immune response system may also be affected by the presence of bifidobacteria. Cell wall fractions of *Bifido infantis* are known to contain active anti-tumor constituents. Meanwhile, healthy populations of beneficial bacteria activate the immune system's macrophages and they become more alert on the job.

Bolstering the body's balance of *Lactobacillus acidophilus* may truly prevent colon cancer. In an experimental crossover study, 21 healthy subjects were given viable lactobacillus cultures with milk or milk without the cultures. The fecal concentration of bacterial enzymes that convert procarcinogens into full-fledged carcinogens was significantly reduced within one month in persons receiving the lactobacillus cultures but not in the group receiving the placebo.[75]

In another study, the authors noted that the link between diet and colon cancer can be explained, in part, by the alteration of fecal bacterial enzyme activity caused by the Western-style diet which is high in beef and saturated fat and low in fiber.[76] Such alterations in microfloral balance can be normalized with prebiotics such as inulin.

Cancer Prevention

BREAST CANCER

Breast cancer is the cause of over six-hundred-thousand deaths yearly worldwide.[77] And forty-six thousand in the United States. The majority of these were among postmenopausal women under seventy: premature death sentences, robbing these women of fifteen to twenty years of life. According to a renowned international authority:

"It is the leading cause of cancer death in women throughout the industrialized world and in many developing countries."[79]

There is a real and significant increase in breast cancer throughout the industrialized nations. Worldwide, one in eleven women in industrialized nations will develop breast cancer.[80] In the United States, from 1950 to 1991, incidence increased fifty-five percent. An even more reliable estimate, including people of color, puts the increase, from only 1973 to 1991, at twenty-four percent.[81] Furthermore, these figures reflect incidence, a more accurate indicator than mortality, which is influenced by a wide range of factors including access to health care.

Fortunately, breast cancer is another malignant disease that friendly bacteria may protect against. For example, in one experimental study on breast cancer, "the growth of both tumor lines was significantly inhibited by supplementing the diet with nondigestible carbohydrates [i.e., inulin]. Such non-toxic dietary treatment appears to be easy and risk-free for patients, applicable as an adjuvant factor in the classical protocols of human cancer therapy."[82]

Lactobacillus inhibits beta-glucuronidase, the fecal bacterial enzyme that prevents the body from detoxifying more potent forms of estrogen (such as estradiol) into less toxic forms (e.g., estriol). Toxic forms of estrogen increase women's risk of breast cancer.[83] Thus, inulin may play an important role in normalizing the gut flora that would help to defuse the most toxic forms of estrogen.

NINE

Diabetes

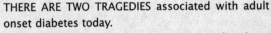

THERE ARE TWO TRAGEDIES associated with adult onset diabetes today.

The first is that by the time a person has been diagnosed with this condition, he or she has most likely already had it several years or longer. Extensive damage to the nervous and circulatory systems and even to their vision may have already occurred.

The second tragedy is that diabetes is striking baby boomers with a vengeance. About six percent of our population presently has diabetes. Many experts believe that percentage will increase significantly as the boomers enter their fifties and sixties. And they say that diet and nutrition will be crucial to helping persons with diabetes maintain their health and reduce their risk of complications.

Adult onset diabetes is a dangerous disease. You should be aware of the risk factors and symptoms.

Inulin (not to be confused with *insulin*) can also help. Inulin has a long history of use for normalizing blood sugar levels. Because inulin is only digested to a negligible extent during its passage through the human mouth, stomach and small intestine, it has no adverse effect on blood glucose levels when ingested orally.

The potential use of inulin as a food for diabetics has been known since the beginning of the 20th century. As early as 1905, inulin was being recommended to diabetics and it was found that among diabetics it was well digested and assimilated even in large doses and through long periods of time. In 1911, it was reported that feeding 40 to 100 grams per day of pure inulin was very beneficial for diabetics. Since then, many more applications have been described in the litera-

CYBER INFO SITE

If you tend to eat too much, are obese and over 40 you're at risk for adult diabetes. If you are more than twenty percent above your ideal weight, over 50 and female, your risk for diabetes is even greater. People with a family history of the disorder are also at higher than normal risk.

Type II (or adult-onset) diabetes accounts for 90 percent of all cases of diabetes, but there are symptoms which are more or less common to all forms of diabetes. Do you ever feel a heaviness in your lower legs, tingling, or suffer nocturnal cramps? Do your fingers sometimes feel alternately numb or tingly? Is your vision deteriorating? Do you suffer leg ulcers? Do you urinate much more than usual, sometimes as often as every hour? Are you often unusually thirsty? And does consuming sweetened beverages increase the amount you urinate and worsen your thirst? Do you often feel extremely tired, weak and apathetic? Is it difficult to get up in the morning? Do you suffer from foot or leg ulcers or varicose veins?

Any of these symptoms, alone or together, means you could be suffering from diabetes. Unfortunately by the time these symptoms appear, it is likely that you've already been suffering from diabetes for several years. That is why it is important *not* to delay seeing your health professional to be sure of the diagnosis or in taking positive steps to improve your overall health.

ture, including inulin-based diabetic bread and pastry and inulin-based diabetic jam. In fact, today inulin is a major ingredient throughout Europe in diabetic foods.

Inulin is the ultimate complex carbohydrate. It is a storage carbohydrate as well as one of the few known soluble fibers. It is the only carbohydrate that extends carbohydrate-derived energy over extended periods without significant increases in blood sugar level and does not require insulin in order to be metabolized. Inulin can help reduce insulin dependencies and requirements as well as provide better blood sugar control. The long-term *Diabetes* energy release which inulin provides not only prevents low blood sugar levels in diabetics but enhances endurance for the normal active individual.

This benefit for diabetics was recently confirmed in the May 11, 2000 *New England Journal of Medicine* when researchers noted a high intake of fiber, particularly of the soluble type (such as inulin), "improves glycemic control, decreases hyperinsulinemia, and lowers plasma lipid concentrations in patients with type 2 diabetes."

Inulin spreads the absorption of carbohydrates over a longer period of time than absorption without inulin. This is important because stretching carbohydrate utilization over periods from two to ten hours delays the pangs of hunger that result from the sugar rush and subsequent low experienced with carbohydrate consumption. For athletes, this capacity increases endurance levels as well. For diabetics, the fact that inulin does not increase blood sugar levels and prevents low blood sugar levels is important in preventing diabetic ketoacidosis and can actually tone down the amount of injected insulin required. Thus, inulin can be of benefit to diabetics, people with a propensity towards diabetes, and normal, active individuals. The importance of inulin to diabetics as a "buffer" for maintaining constant blood sugar levels and to athletes and normal individuals as an "energy sustainer," providing endurance, cannot be stressed enough.

TEN

Inulin & Weight Control

VERY RECENTLY, I DISCOVERED a Jerusalem artichoke fiber-based candy called **Inu-lean™**. Not only does it taste great, I've begun seeing excellent results when my patients use it as a non-stimulating appetite suppressant. Because Jerusalem artichoke fiber has none of the toxicity problems associated with ma huang- and caffeine-containing appetite suppressants, it could be an important dieter's aid. After all, we all know that a high-fiber diet tends to suppress the appetite.

Many of my patients have confided that Inu-lean is one of the best tasting "health candies" they've ever had the pleasure of wrapping their taste buds around. Imagine a candy so sweet, yet so healthy—one that fills your tummy with hunger-inhibiting Jerusalem artichoke fiber, provides energy, and helps to populate your gastrointestinal tract with immune-supportive beneficial bacteria. That's Inu-lean. And kids loves Inu-lean, too. It's a great "candy" for everyone. I'd much rather see my youngest child munching Inu-lean chewables than sugar-laden candy bars.

Inu-lean chewables are great for kids, dieters—and anyone with a sweet tooth, yet who has yen for health. Each Inu-lean tablet provides almost one gram of coveted Jerusalem artichoke fiber and only about six calories—plus it has a tasty chocolate mint flavor.

Give 'em to your children for a healthy treat. And if you're hungry and dieting, chew three or four to quench your appetite without the need for artificial stimulants.

One warning. They taste so good, three or four may not be enough. But even if you munch a baker's dozen, you're still only at about 78 calories and that's a whole lot less calories and a lot more health than a check-out line candy bar!

Plus, I think you'll find, as have my patients, that with Inu-lean chewables you can easily avoid excessive snacking between meals or before bedtime. If your problem is eating between meals or eating industrial-sized portions at lunch or dinner, try regularly consuming three to five Inu-lean chewables between meals. I think you'll be pleasantly surprised at your newly discovered appetite control.

ELEVEN

Inulin vs. Probiotics

THERE ARE MANY PRODUCTS SOLD TODAY as dietary supplements that are alleged to provide cultures of live friendly bacteria. These products that claim to provide live bacterial culture are called *probiotics*. In contrast, inulin is a *pre*biotic and provides food or "fertilizer" to the bacterial colonies already residing in your gastrointestinal tract.

Naturally, you may be wondering whether inulin holds any advantages over probiotics or whether the two should be used simultaneously.

Both prebiotics and probiotics can be very helpful.

But that said, I have real concerns with probiotic formulas sold today.

First, to insure that friendly strains of bacteria in dietary supplements actually provide their therapeutic benefits, they must implant and propagate rapidly once in the gut to avoid being eliminated entirely. Thus, the bacteria must be able to survive the high stomach acidity and then actually adhere to intestinal epithelial cells even in the presence of high levels of bile salts.

It should be recognized that being live organisms, bacteria in such preparations do not readily tolerate the harsh acidic environment in the stomach, and may be totally compromised by the time they reach the intestine. Even those bacteria that do survive the strong stomach acid may be utterly compromised as to not be able to compete in the intestine for food and energy. Thus, they cannot colonize the intestine.

A second serious problem is that many such products researchers have tested do not provide live cultures—even though they claim to do so on their labels. That is, they lack stability. By the time, these organisms have been subjected to the rigors of handling, transportation, changes in temperature and shelf storage most of them have died.

In one study, seventy to eighty percent of samples did not measure up to label claims. In fact, fifty percent did not even have ten percent of the claimed number of live microorganisms. Some products did not even have the strains of bacteria that they claimed to have. One product had *Streptococcus lactis* and several samples had pathogenic organisms present. These reflect not only the observations of my own research but of previously published papers from leading experts in the field of microbiology.[84, 85]

Inulin, on the other hand, simply feeds the bacteria that are already in the gastrointestinal tract. There is nothing to keep it from working. We know it works. We do not need to worry about viability.

That said, there are some excellent prebiotic formulas. What's more, both probiotics and prebiotics may be used together.

But the difficulty is in finding products with live cultures. I hope that with publication of such data on the quality of probiotic products in the near future, consumers will be able to make such selections.

Until that time, I advise consumers to use prebiotics such as inulin and to consider the use of probiotics as an option, preferring quality formulas from companies such as Enzymatic Therapy and Metagenics.

TWELVE

Enhancing the Healing Response

IN THIS BOOK, I HAVE ENDEAVORED to open up your mind to a new pathway of healing and a way to make your doctors' antibiotics work better to benefit your health.

Whether called Energy, Vital Force, or even Karma, there is a Life Essence that must be protected. Look around you. You watch people get sick by literally giving their life away. They make bad choices and just like a car leaking oil, they let their energy leak away. Also note, that when a person is healthy, they have ample vital force. So much so, that they can boost yours with a hug. *Regular use of inulin can contribute to your life force.*

Make healthy choices!

Preserving natural and adequate movement of Vital Force is essential. Moving our bodies assures enough blood and oxygen. Just as blood flows in one direction, so does energy.

Homeostasis is a dynamic ever-changing move toward balance in which your body is involved. Stasis, on the other hand, is stagnation. Your body will make every effort to preserve homeostasis and avoid stasis. Inulin can help your body to achieve the dynamic balance of homeostasis.

Stasis is a cardinal concept for explaining the etiology of illnesses. If you clog the system, sickness ensues. Inulin literally helps to unclog your system.

Your body responds automatically to most conditions. It does so at a cellular level. We are used to talking about reflexes and the autonomic nervous system. Why is it so difficult to admit that our gastrointestinal system is also part of our nervous system?

Again, inulin will help to care for your second brain, your gut. Perhaps, the toughest concept to accept is that your brain is in equilibrium with our cells. Our mind (consciousness—the holder of beliefs), as we understand it, relays back and forth what happens both on a cellular level and a behavioral level. For example, we know that bitterness causes depression and that depression is linked to higher incidence of disease. We also know that love within a stable long-term relationship leads to longer life and better health. Disease is a consequence of the loss of equilibrium.

Environment induces potential genetic expression. In a safe environment, illness will not occur. The physical, emotional, mental, and spiritual body are protected in such environments. The emphasis on milieu for maintaining health and enhancing healing cannot be overstated. It takes a lot of love and a loving family to enjoy health.

Toxins exist internally and externally and as chemicals and emotions. Our physical and energetic body must shield and actively defend itself. Here, inulin is very helpful. An arsenal of defenders must be present, trained and ready to act. Any threat to the physical and energetic body must be met with active forces. A healthy immune system is essential, as is belief in God. Vitamins, minerals, herbs, antioxidants, enzymes and fiber are key defenders—especially inulin. Maintain supernutrient status.

Accept your healthy blessings from the Jerusalem artichoke!

A Guide to the Players: A Glossary of Gastrointestinal Ecology

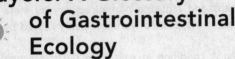

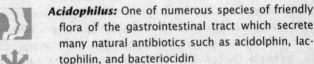

Acidophilus: One of numerous species of friendly flora of the gastrointestinal tract which secrete many natural antibiotics such as acidolphin, lactophilin, and bacteriocidin

Aerobe: Any of a number of bacteria that require oxygen in the environment to grow and multiply.

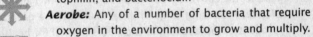

Anaerobe or Anaerobic: Any of a number of bacteria that grow in the absence of oxygen. Many bacteria grow only in the absence of oxygen and are said to be anaerobic bacteria.

Antibiotic: Any of a large of group of chemical substances such as penicillin and streptomycin that are produced by various microorganisms and fungi and have the capacity in dilute solutions to inhibit the growth of or to destroy bacteria and other microorganisms and are used in the treatment of infectious diseases.

Bacteriocidal: Used to refer to substances that kill bacteria directly.

Bacterostatic: Antibiotics that kill bacteria indirectly by interfering with cell wall synthesis or other parts of the metabolism necessary for bacterial growth.

Bifidobacterium: A family of anaerobic friendly bacteria that are found in the alimentary tract and feces of infants and older people. These are the most common species found in human infants and help confer protection against infection. One particular strain *Bifidus infantis* is used therapeutically for treatment of infant diarrhea.

Biota: The animal, plants or fungi of a region, including of the body.

Chronic Fatigue Syndrome: Fatigue lasting greater than six months and reducing normal activity by more than fifty percent. Associated with, and likely caused by, dysbiosis.

Dysbiosis: A condition in which the gastrointestinal system's bacterial populations become disturbed.

Ecosystem: A system formed by the interaction of a community of organisms with its environment.

Fermentation: Any of a group of living organisms as yeasts, molds, and certain bacteria, that cause a chemical change in the absence of oxygen that yields energy; for example, the conversion of grape sugar into ethyl alcohol.

Flatulence: Producing of gastrointestinal gas, the gaseous byproduct of metabolism of food. It is normal for healthy persons to pass small amounts of gas some 14 to 23 times daily.

Flora: The aggregate of bacteria, fungi and other microorganisms occurring on or within the body, as in *intestinal flora*.

Fructooligosaccharide: Complex groups of sugar molecules containing fructose and chains of glycogen also known as FOS. These substances are non-absorbable and difficult for the body to digest, but act as food to friendly flora of the gastrointestinal tract. Inulin is an FOS.

Fungi: A group of spore-forming organisms that, when allowed to grow uncontrollably, compete with normal flora, and can cause disease and seriously compromise homeostasis.

Inulin: A leading prebiotic long used in Europe and now available in the United States. Used simultaneously with antibiotics to foster growth of beneficial bacteria whose populations may have been harmed or destroyed by the broad-spectrum effect of antibiotics.

Irritable Bowel Syndrome: Also known as IBS, this is a common functional disorder of the intestines estimated to affect five million Americans. The cause of IBS is not yet known. Doctors refer to IBS as a functional disorder because there is no sign of disease when the colon is examined. But functional, in this case, means "dysfunctional." Doctors believe that people with IBS experience abnormal patterns of colonic movement and absorption capabilities. The IBS colon is highly sensitive, overreacting to any stimuli such as gas, stress, or eating high-fat or fiber-rich foods.

Lactobacillus: Any of various anaerobic bacteria of the family *Lactobacillus* capable of breaking down carbohydrates to form lactic acid. With many health-promoting properties, lactobacillis help to displace toxin-producing pathogenic strains. They also aid in the prevention of cancer

Leaky Gut Syndrome: A condition where the membranes of the gut are highly permeable allowing large, allergenic molecules to pass into the systemic circulation and cause disease.

Listeria: An infectious disease, often deadly to infants and elderly.

Macrophages: The white blood cells of the immune system responsible for protection against bacteria and other pathogens. The first line of defense of the immune system.

Natural Killer Cells: Cells of the immune system that attack cancerous and other damaged cells.

Peristalsis: Progressive waves of involuntary muscle contractions and relaxations that move matter along certain tube-like structures of the body, as in the case of ingested food along the alimentary canal.

Prebiotic: Any substance that beneficially feeds the bacteria in the intestinal tract and stimulates growth of friendly bacteria. A prebiotic may be thought of as "fertilizer" for the good bacteria in the gastrointestinal tract. Think of inulin as a prebiotic.

Probiotic: Whereas an antibiotic kills bacteria, often indiscriminately, a probiotic supports life and provides bacteria to the gastrointestinal tract. Probiotic formulas usually contain various species of lactobacillus and bifidobacteria.

Protozoa: Small, parasitic organisms that can cause disease, technically protozoa are not bacteria because of their structure, although fully capable of causing major infectious illness such as syphilis and Lyme disease.

Salubrity: State of enviable health achieved by adhering to principles of responsible personal hygiene.

Steroid: There are two major classes of corticosteroids, commonly called "steroids." Those derived from cortisone are known as anti-inflammatory steroids and are very potent anti-inflammatory agents, but known to have multiple long term deleterious side effects. When given for prolonged periods and in high doses, they will cause the overgrowth of opportunistic infectious microorganisms such as yeast, most notably candida. (The other class of steroids, known as anabolic steroids, are often used by athletes to bulk up.)

Synergy: An interaction of elements that, when combined, produce a total effect greater than the sum of the individual elements.

Triglycerides: The form in which fat exists in meats, cheese, fish, nuts, vegetable oils, and the greasy layer on the surface of soup stocks or in a pan in which bacon has been fried. In a healthy person, triglycerides and other fatty substances are normally moved into the liver and into storage cells to provide energy for later use.

Additional Readings

Gershon, M. *The Second Brain—Our Gut*,
New York: HarperCollins, 1998

Richter, J.E. *Medical Management for
Gastroesophageal Reflux Disease*—1995.
The American College of Gastroenterology Annual
Postgraduate Course. New York, 1995: 1a-55-61.

Sachs G., Prinz, K.C., & Hersey, J.S. *Acid-Related
Disorders: Mystery to Mechanism, Mechanism to
Management*. Florida: Sushu Publishing, Inc. 1995: 71-80.

The following organizations also distribute materials and offer
support programs for patients with digestive diseases:

American Liver Foundation
1425 Pompton Avenue
Cedar Grove, NJ 07009
(201) 256-2550

Crohn's & Colitis Foundation of America, Inc.
386 Park Avenue South, 17th Floor
New York, NY 10016-8804
(800) 932-2423
(212) 685-3440

International Foundation for Bowel Dysfunction
P.O. Box 17864
Milwaukee, WI 53217
(414) 241-9479

IMPORTANT REPORT AVAILABLE
ON CHILDREN'S VITAMINS

To obtain our special investigative report on children's vitamins in which we rate many of the leading brands and discuss how inulin works in other ways to improve children's health, please send $2.95 to Freedom Press, 1801 Chart Trail, Topanga, CA 90290 or visit our website at www.freedompressonline.com.

FREE TRIAL SUBSCRIPTION TO
THE DOCTORS' PRESCRIPTION
FOR HEALTHY LIVING

Send us your name and address for a free trial subscription to **The Doctors' Prescription for Healthy Living**. Just write or fax: **The Doctors' Prescription for Healthy Living**, 1801 Chart Trail, Topanga, CA 90290 or fax to (310) 455-8962 or (310) 455-3203.

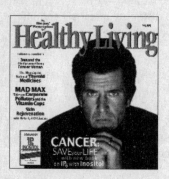

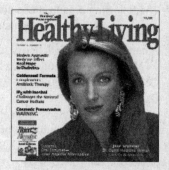

Resources

AT THIS TIME, THERE IS ONLY ONE BRAND of Jerusalem artichoke fiber is available in the United States. It is known as InuFlora™ when sold as a powder and as Inu-lean™ when purchased as delicious chewables.

Both InuFlora and Inu-lean chewables are available at health food stores, natural product supermarkets, pharmacies, from health professionals, by mail-order, and through the worldwide web.

Many consumers prefer the powder form to the pills because inulin mixes so easily with their favorite juice and has a sweet pleasant taste.

However, many children absolutely love Inu-lean chewables and eat them like "candy." The chewables are also excellent for dieters who wish to stave off sugar cravings with a healthy "candy" that supplies them with minimal calories and maximum fiber.

For more information on InuFlora and Inu-Lean in retail outlets, contact Marlyn Neutraceuticals/Naturally Vitamins, 14851 North Scottsdale Road, Scottsdale, AZ 85254, (800) 899-4499. Web site: www.naturallyvitamins.com.

To purchase InuFlora or Inu-Lean by mail, on the internet or by convenient use of the phone, contact AgeSmart, 22287 Mulholland Highway, Calabasas, CA 91302, 1-877-243-7627 (AGE-SMART).

For additional inulin information and its other exciting applications in health and medicine, visit www.freedompressonline.com.

References

1 Glissen, G. *Immunität und Infektion*, 1980; 8: 79-88.
2 Cohen, M., "Epidemiology of drug resistance: implications for a post-antibiotic era." *Science*, 1992; 257: 1050.
3 Reuters. "Drug resistant bacteria found in rural U.S.," September 30, 1999.
4 Pignataa C, Budillon G, Monaco G, Nani E, Cuomo R, Parrilli G, and Ciccimarra F. "Jejunal bacterial overgrowth and intestinal permeability in children with immunodeficiency syndromes." *Gut* 1990; 31: 879-882.
5 Csordas A. Toxicology of butyrate and short-chain fatty acids. In: *Role of Gut Bacteria in Human Toxicology and Pharmacology*, M. Hill, ed., Bristol: Taylor & Francis Inc., 1995, p. 286.
6 Hunnisett A., et al. "Gut fermentation (or the autobrewery) syndrome: a new clinical test with initial observations and discussion of clinical and biochemical implications." *J Nut Med* 1:33-38 (1990).
7 The diseases and conditions discussed in this overview are covered in greater detail by fact sheets and information packets. The statistics reported in this fact sheet come from *Digestive Diseases in the United States: Epidemiology and Impact*, edited by James Everhart, M.D., MPH., NIH Publication No. 94-1447. For copies of fact sheets, information packets, or the *Digestive Diseases in the U.S.*, you may contact the National Digestive Diseases Information Clearinghouse (NDDIC), 2 Information Way, Bethesda, MD 20892-3570.
8 Melñikova V.M., et al. "Problems in drug prevention and treatment of endogenous infection and dysbacteriosis." *Vestn Ross Akad Med Nauk*, 1997; (3):26-9.

9 Eaton K.K., et al. "Abnormal gut fermentation: Laboratory studies reveal deficiency of B vitamins, zinc, and magnesium." *J Nutr Biochem* 4 (Nov): 635-637 (1993).

10 Zoppi, G., et al. "The intestinal ecosystem in chronic functional constipation." *Acta Paediatr*, 1998; 87(8):836-841.

11 Gorman, C. "Healthy germs." *Time*, December 28, 1998-January 4, 1999: 197.

12 Vanderhoof, J.A. & Young, R.J. "Use of probiotics in childhood gastrointestinal disorders." *Pediatr Gastroenterol Nutr*, 1998; 27(3):323-32.

13 Wang, X. & Gibson, G.B. "Effects of the *in vitro* fermentation of oligofructose and inulin by bacteria growing in the human large intestine." *Journal of Applied Bacteriology*, 1993; 75(4): 373-380.

14 Brandt, L. "New inulin offers high performance." *Prepared Foods*, May 1998.

15 Moshfegh, A.J., et al. "Presence of inulin and oligofructose in the diets of Americans." *Journal of Nutrition*, 1999; 129(7 Suppl): 1407S-1411S.

16 Heinerman, J. *Super Immune Power Through a Healthy Intestinal Tract*. Québec, Canada: DynaMark Corporation Inc., 1998.

17 Gibson, G.R., et al. "Selective stimulation of bifidobacteria in the human colon by oligofructose and inulin." *Gastroenterology*, 1995; 108(4): 975-982.

18 Oli, M.W., et al. "Evaluation of fructooligosaccharide supplementation of oral electrolyte solutions for treatment of diarrhea: recovery of the intestinal bacteria." *Dig Dis Sci*, 1998; 43(1):138-147.

19 Bouhnik, Y., et al. "Effects of bifidobacterium sp fermented milk ingested with or without inulin on colonic bifidobacteria and enzymatic activities in healthy humans." *Eur J Clin Nutr*, 1996; 50(4): 269-273.

20 Kleesen, N., et al. "Effects of inulin and lactose on fecal microflora, microbial activity, and bowel habit in elderly constipated persons." *Am J Clin Nutr*, 1997; 65(5): 1397-1402.

21 Fukata, T., et al. "Inhibitory effects of competitive exclusion and fructooligosaccharide, singly and in combination, on Salmonella colonization of chicks." *J Food Prot*, 1999; 62(3): 229-233.

References

22 D'Angelo, G., et al. "Probiotics in childhood." *Minerva Pediatr*, 1998; 50(5):163-73.

23 "The poop on probiotics." *Natural Foods Merchandiser*, January 1999; 55.

24 Niv, M., et al. "Yogurt in the treatment of infantile diarrhea." *Clin. Ped.*, 1963; 2: 407-411.

25 Kleessen, B., et al. "Effects of inulin and lactose on fecal microflora, microbial activity, and bowel habit in elderly constipated persons." *Am J Clin Nutr* 1997; 65(5): 1397-1402.

26 *Lancet general Advertiser*, September 21, 1957.

27 Rettger, L.F., et al. *Lactobacillus acidophilus. Its therapeutic application*. New Haven: Yale University Press, 1935.

28 Kopeloff, N. "Clinical results obtained with bacillus acidophilus." *Arch Int Med*, 1924; 33: 47.

29 Weinstein, L.,et al. "Therapeutic application of acidophilus milk in simple constipation." *Arch Int Med*, 1933; 52: 384.

30 Fernandes, C.F., et al. "Control of diarrhea by lactobacilli." *J Appl Nutr*, 1988; 40: 32-43.

31 Fernandes, C.F., et al. "Effect of nutrient media and bile salts on growth and antimicrobial activity of *L. acidophilus*." *J Dairy Sci*, 1988; 71: 3222-3228.

32 Thorwald, J. *Science and Secrets of Early Medicine*. New York: Harcourt, Brace & World, 1963, pp. 84-87.

33 Schiffin, E., et al. *American Journal of Clinical Nutrition*, 1997; 66: 515S-520S.

34 Shahani, K.M., et al. *Cultured Dairy Products Journal*, 1977; 12: 8-11.

35 Shahani, K.M. & Ayebo, A.D. "Role of dietary lactobacilli in gastrointestinal microecology." *American Journal of Clinical Nutrition*, 1980; 33: 2448-2457.

36 Shahani, K.M., et al. "Antibiotic acidophilus and the process for preparing the same." U.S. Patent 3,689,640, September 5, 1972.

37 Reddy, G.V., et al. "Natural antibiotic activity of *L. acidophilus* and *bulgaricus*. III. Production and partial purification of bulgarican from *L. bulgaricus*." *Cultured Dairy Pro J*, 1983; 18(2): 15-19.

38 "Effect of lactobacillus immunotherapy on genital infections in women (Solco/Gynatren)." *Geburtshilfe Fraunheilkd*, 1984; 44(5): 311-314.

39 Fredricsson, B., et al. "Gardnerella-associated vaginitis and anerobic bacteria." *Gynecol. Obstet. Invest.*, 1984; 17(5): 236-241.

40 Spiegel, C.A., et al. "Diagnosis of bacterial vaginosis by direct gram stain of vaginal fluid." *J. Clin. Microbiol.*, 1983; 18(1): 170-177.

41 Spiegel, C.A., et al. "Anaerobic bacteria in nonspecific vaginitis." *The New England Journal of Medicine*, 1980; 303(11): 601-607.

42 Mintz, M. "FDA evaluates link between cancer, drug." *The Washington Post*, January 21, 1976.

43 Rustia, M. & Shubik, P. "Experimental induction of hepatomas, mammary tumors, and other tumors with metronidazole in nonbred Sas:MRC(WI)BR rats." *Journal of the National Cancer Institute*, 1979; 63: 863-868.

44 Cavaliere, A., et al. "Induction of mammary tumors with metronidazole in female Sprague-Dawley rats." *Tumori*, 1984; 70: 307-311.

45 Danielson, D.A., et al. "Metronidazole and cancer." *Journal of the American Medical Association*, 1982; 247(18): 2498-2499

46 Beard, C.M., et al. "Lack of evidence for cancer due to use of metronidazole." *The New England Journal of Medicine*, 1979; 301(10): 519-522.

47 Karkut, G. "[Effect of lactobacillus immunotherapy on genital infections in women (Solco Trichovac/Gynatren)." *Geburtshilfe Fraunheilkd*, 1984; 44(5): 311-314.

48 Litschgi, M.S., et al. "Effectiveness of a lactobacillus vaccine on trichomonas infections in women. Preliminary results." *Fortschr. Med.*, 1980; 98(41): 1624-1627.

49 Will, T.E. "Lactobacillus overgrowth for treatment of moniliary vulvovaginitis." Letter to the editor. *Lancet*, 1979; 2: 482.

50 Chandan, R.C.Y., et al. "Competitive exclusion of uropathogens from human uroepithelial cells by Lactobacillus." *Infect Immun*, 1985; 47: 84-89.

51 Kuvaeva, I., et al. "The microecology of the gastrointestinal tract and the immunological status under food allergy." *Nahrung*, 1984; 28(6-7): 689-693.

52 Galbraith, R.A. & Michnovicz, J.J. "The effects of cimetidine on the oxidative metabolism of estradiol." *The New England Journal of Medicine*, 1989; 321(5): 269-274.

53 Smedley, H.M. "Malignant breast change in man given two drugs associated with breast hyperplasia." *The Lancet*, 1981; 2: 638-639.

References

54 Lee, H., et al. "Factors affecting the protein quality of yogurt and acidophilus milk." *J Dairy Sci*, 1988; 71: 3203-3214.

55 Fernandes, C.F., et al. "Therapeutic role of dietary alctobacilli and lactobacillic fermented dairy products." *FEMS Microbiol Rev*, 1987; 46: 343-356.

56 Fernandes, C.F. & Shahani, K.M. "Lactose intolerance and its modulation with Lactobacilli and other microbial supplements." *J Appl Nutr*, 1989; 41: 50-64.

57 Gilliland, S.E. "Health and nutritional benefits from lactic acid bacteria." *FEMS Microbial Rev*, 1990; 87: 175-188.

58 *Lancet General Advertiser*, September 21, 1957.

59 Manning, A.P., et al. "Wheat fibre and irritable bowel syndrome: A controlled trial." *Lancet*, 1977; 2: 417.

60 Fielding, J., et al. "Different dietary fibre formulations and the irritable bowel syndrome." *Irish J. Med. Sci.*, 1984; 153: 178-180.

61 Ohta, A., et al. "Dietary fructooligosaccharides prevent osteopenia after gastrectomy in rats." *J Nutr*, 1998; 128(1):106-10.

62 Morohashi, T., et al. "True calcium absorption in the intestine is enhanced by fructooligosaccharide feeding in rats." *J Nutr*, 1998; 128(10):1815-1818.

63 Shahani, K.M. & Ayebo, A.D. "Role of dietary lactobacilli in gastrointestinal microecology." *Proc VI International Symposium Intestinal Microecology. Am J Clin Nutr*, 1980; 33: 2448-2457.

64 Rao, D. & Shahani, K.M. "Vitamin content of culture dairy products." *Cultured Dairy Prod*, 1987; 22(1): 6-10.

65 Jeppesen, J., et al. "Triglyceride concentration and ischemic heart disease: an eight-year follow-up in the Copenhagen Male Study." *Circulation*, 1998 97: 1029-1036.

66 Roberfroid, M.B. "Functional effects of food components and the gastrointestinal system: chicory fructooligosaccharides." *Nutr Rev*, 1996; 54(11 Pt 2):S38-42.

67 Williams, C.M. "Effects of inulin on lipid parameters in humans." *J Nutr*, 1999; 129(7 Suppl):1471S-1473S.

68 Davidson, M.H. & Maki, K.C. "Effects of dietary inulin on serum lipids." *Journal of Nutrition*, 1999 129(7 Suppl): 1474S-1477S.

69 Liebman, B. "Diet & disease: the story so far." *Nutrition Action Health Letter*, 1999; 26(10): 1, 3-9.

70 Fernandes, C.F., et al. "Mode of tumor suppression by *Lactobacillus acidophilus*." *J Nutr Medicine*, 1991; 2: 25-34.

71 Bottazzi, V., et al. "Properta antitumorali dei batteri latticie degl. Alimenti fermentati con batteri lacttici." *Il Latte*, 1985; 10: 873-879.

72 Podell, R.N. "Bacteria that strengthen the immune system." *Health & Nutrition Breakthroughs*, February 1998: 12.

73 Reddy, B.S. "Possible mechanisms by which pro- and prebiotics influence colon carcinogenesis and tumor growth." *Journal of Nutrition*, 1999; 129(7 Suppl): 1478S-1482S.

74 Lee, H., et al. "Anticarcinogenic effect of *Lactobacillus acidophilus* on N-nitrosobis (2-oxopropyl)amine induced colon tumor in rats." *J Appl Nutr*, 1996; 48: 59-66.

75 Goldin, B.R. & Gorbach, S.L. "The effect of milk and lactobacillus feeding on human intestinal bacteria enzyme activity." *American Journal of Clinical Nutrition*, 1984; 39: 756-761.

76 Gorbach, S.L. "The intestinal microflora and its colon cancer connection." *Infection*, 1982; 10(6): 379-384.

77 Kohlmeier, L., et al. "Lifestyle trends in worldwide breast cancer rates." *Trends in Cancer Mortality in Industrial Countries*. New York, NY: The New York Academy of Sciences, 1990.

78 Ibid.

79 Ibid.

80 Ibid.

81 National Cancer Institute Surveillance, Epidemiology and End Results.

82 Taper, H.S. & Roberfroid, M. "Influence of inulin and oligofructose on breast cancer and tumor growth." *Journal of Nutrition*, 1999; 129 (7 Suppl): 1488S-1491S.

83 Goldin, B. & Gorsbach, S. "The effect of milk and lactobacillus feeding on human intestinal bacterial enzyme activity." *American Journal of Clinical Nutrition*, 1984; 39: 756-761.

84 Gilliland, S.E. & Speck, M.L. "Enumeration and identity of lactobacilli in dietary products." *J Food Prot*, 1977; 40: 760-762.

85 Brenna, M., et al. "Prevalence of viable lactobacillus acidophilus in dried commercial products." *J Food Prot*, 1983; 46: 887-892.

References

The Author

MICHAEL W. LOES, M.D., M.D.(H.), is currently the director of the Arizona Pain Institute, a division of the University of Arizona's Integrative Program in anesthesiology. He completed medical school at the University of Minnesota, followed by a fellowship in clinical pharmacology. His residency training was in internal medicine at the University of Arizona in Tucson. He is board certified in internal medicine with subspecialty board certifications in pain medicine and management, alcohol and chemical dependency, acupuncture, clinical hypnosis, homeopathy and disability medicine. He is a faculty assistant professor at the University of Arizona Health Science Center, Tucson, and a former faculty consultant to the Mayo Clinic Scottsdale Pain Center. He has helped thousands of chronic pain patients over the years to regain their health by enhancing their bodies' healing powers, using many of the techniques detailed in this book, including Wobenzym N. Dr. Loes is co-author of *Arthritis: The Doctors' Cure* (Keats Publishing 1998), *The Aspirin Alternative* (Freedom Press 1999), and *The Non-drug European Secret to Healing Sports Injuries Naturally* (Freedom Press 1999).